The 50+ Intermittent Fasting Plan

A Comprehensive Guide to Intermittent Fasting for Men and Women Over 50 - Achieve Weight Loss, Fitness, and Wellness with a 21-Day Meal Plan

BY
ADEEL ANJUM

CONTENTS

INTRODUCTION   1

Chapter 01
Understanding Intermittent Fasting 8
Chapter 02
The Benefits of Intermittent Fasting for the 50+ Population 15
Chapter 03
The Science Behind Intermittent Fasting 27
Chapter 04
Getting Started with Intermittent Fasting 35
Chapter 05
Customizing Your Fasting Plan 44
Chapter 06
Nutrition and Intermittent Fasting 53
Chapter 07
Overcoming Common Challenges 62
Chapter 08
Intermittent Fasting and Exercise 71
Chapter 09
Mental and Emotional Well-being 81
Chapter 10
Monitoring Your Progress 90
Chapter 11
Special Considerations for Women Over 50 100
Chapter 12
Special Considerations for Men Over 50 108
Chapter 13
Intermittent Fasting and Chronic Conditions 119

Chapter 14
Long-term Sustainability 133
Chapter 15
The 21-Day Meal Plan 145

CONCLUSION   **152**

INTRODUCTION

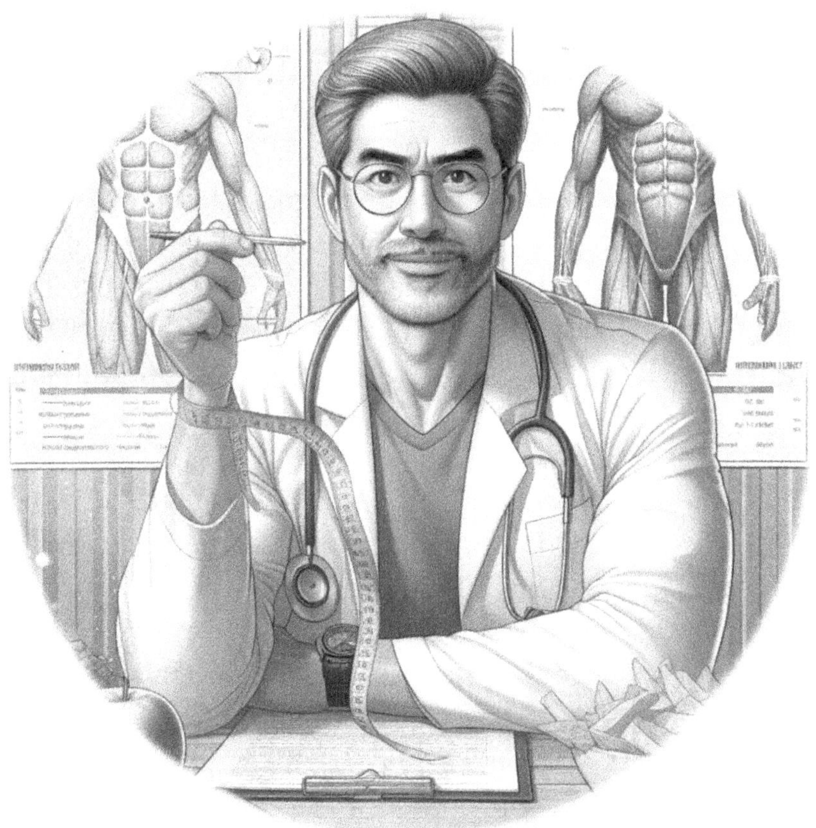

Reaching the milestone of 50 is a significant moment in anyone's life. It marks a period where we reflect on our health and wellness more than ever before. As we age, our bodies undergo changes, and it becomes increasingly important to prioritize our well-being. In this introduction, we'll explore the importance of maintaining health and wellness after 50 and introduce you to the transformative power of intermittent fasting.

Importance of Maintaining Health and Wellness After 50

Entering the fifth decade of life brings with it a host of changes, both physically and mentally. Our metabolism slows down, muscle mass decreases, and our bodies become more susceptible to chronic diseases. However, it's crucial to understand that aging doesn't equate to a decline in health. With the right lifestyle choices, we can not only maintain but improve our overall well-being well into our later years.

After the age of 50, our bodies become more vulnerable to conditions such as heart disease, diabetes, osteoporosis, and certain types of cancer. This is partly due to factors like hormonal changes, decreased muscle mass, and a slower metabolism. However, while genetics play a role, lifestyle choices such as diet, exercise, and stress management also significantly impact our health outcomes.

Moreover, maintaining our health becomes increasingly important as we age because it directly affects our quality of life. We want to enjoy our golden years to the fullest, spending time with loved ones, pursuing hobbies, and traveling. However, poor health can limit our ability to do so, robbing us of the joy and freedom we deserve.

Fortunately, it's never too late to take control of our health and make positive changes. By adopting a holistic approach that encompasses nutrition, physical activity, stress management, and social connection, we can not only extend our lifespan but also improve our vitality and well-being.

Overview of Intermittent Fasting and Its Benefits

Intermittent fasting (IF) has gained significant popularity in recent years, and for good reason. It's not just another fad diet; it's a lifestyle approach backed by science and proven to offer a myriad of health benefits. IF involves cycling between periods of eating and fasting, and it has been linked to weight loss, improved metabolic health, enhanced cognitive function, and longevity.

At its core, intermittent fasting is about changing when you eat rather than what you eat. By incorporating periods of fasting into your routine, you give your body a chance to rest and repair, leading to a wide range of positive effects on both physical and mental health.

One of the key benefits of intermittent fasting is its ability to promote weight loss and fat loss. By restricting the window of time during which you eat, you naturally consume fewer calories, leading to a caloric deficit that can result in weight loss over time. Additionally, fasting triggers hormonal changes that promote fat burning and preserve lean muscle mass, further enhancing your body composition.

Beyond weight loss, intermittent fasting has been shown to improve metabolic health markers such as insulin sensitivity, blood sugar levels, and cholesterol levels. This can reduce the risk of developing chronic diseases such as type 2 diabetes, heart disease, and metabolic syndrome.

Furthermore, intermittent fasting has profound effects on brain health and cognitive function. Studies have demonstrated that fasting can increase the production of brain-derived neurotrophic factor (BDNF), a protein that promotes the growth and survival of neurons. This can enhance memory, learning, and mood, while also reducing the risk of neurodegenerative diseases such as Alzheimer's and Parkinson's.

In addition to these physical and mental health benefits, intermittent fasting has been shown to increase longevity and promote cellular repair processes known as autophagy. This can help protect against age-related decline and extend lifespan in various organisms, including humans.

Overall, intermittent fasting offers a holistic approach to health and wellness that goes beyond just weight loss. By incorporating fasting into your routine, you can optimize your metabolism, support your brain health, and increase your longevity, allowing you to thrive well into your later years.

Personal Stories and Testimonials from Individuals Over 50

Nothing is more inspiring than hearing real-life success stories. Throughout this book, we'll share personal anecdotes and testimonials from individuals over 50 who have embraced intermittent fasting and experienced remarkable transformations. These stories serve as a reminder that age is just a number, and it's never too late to take control of your health and redefine your life.

Imagine Jane, a 55-year-old woman who struggled with her weight and energy levels for years. Despite trying countless diets and exercise programs, she couldn't seem to find a sustainable solution. However, after discovering intermittent fasting, everything changed. By simply adjusting the timing of her meals, Jane was able to effortlessly shed excess pounds, boost her energy, and regain her confidence. Today, she feels better than ever and is grateful for the newfound sense of freedom and vitality that intermittent fasting has given her.

Then there's Mike, a 60-year-old man who was diagnosed with type 2 diabetes and hypertension. Faced with the prospect of a lifetime of medication and declining health, he knew he needed to make a change. That's when he stumbled upon intermittent fasting and decided to give it a try. Within weeks, Mike saw dramatic improvements in his blood sugar levels, blood pressure, and overall health. Today, he's medication-free and feels like a new man, thanks to the power of intermittent fasting.

These are just two examples of the countless individuals who have transformed their lives through intermittent fasting. Whether you're looking to lose weight, reverse chronic disease, or simply feel better overall, intermittent fasting can help you achieve your goals and live your best life.

The Structure and Purpose of the Book

"The 50+ Intermittent Fasting Plan" is designed to be your comprehensive guide to intermittent fasting tailored specifically for men and women over 50. We've structured the book in a way that provides you with all the tools, knowledge, and support you need to embark on your IF journey successfully. From understanding the fundamentals to implementing a 21-day meal plan, we've got you covered every step of the way.

How to Use This Guide Effectively

We understand that starting something new can be daunting, especially when it comes to your health. That's why we've included practical tips and guidance on how to navigate this book effectively. Whether you're a complete beginner or someone familiar with intermittent fasting, we've tailored the information in a way that's easy to understand and implement. So, grab a pen, take notes, and let's embark on this journey together.

Encouragement and Motivation to Start the Journey

Embarking on a new health journey can be intimidating, but it's important to remember that you're not alone. We're here to support and encourage you every step of the way. Whether you're looking to shed a few pounds, improve your energy levels, or simply feel better overall, intermittent fasting can help you achieve your goals. So, let's embrace this opportunity to prioritize our health and wellness as we enter this exciting new chapter of life.

As we dive deeper into the world of intermittent fasting, remember that the journey is just as important as the destination. By taking small, consistent steps toward your goals and staying committed to your health, you have the power to transform your life in ways you never thought possible. So, let's set our intentions, take action, and make the most of this incredible opportunity to reclaim our health and vitality.

Chapter 01

Understanding Intermittent Fasting

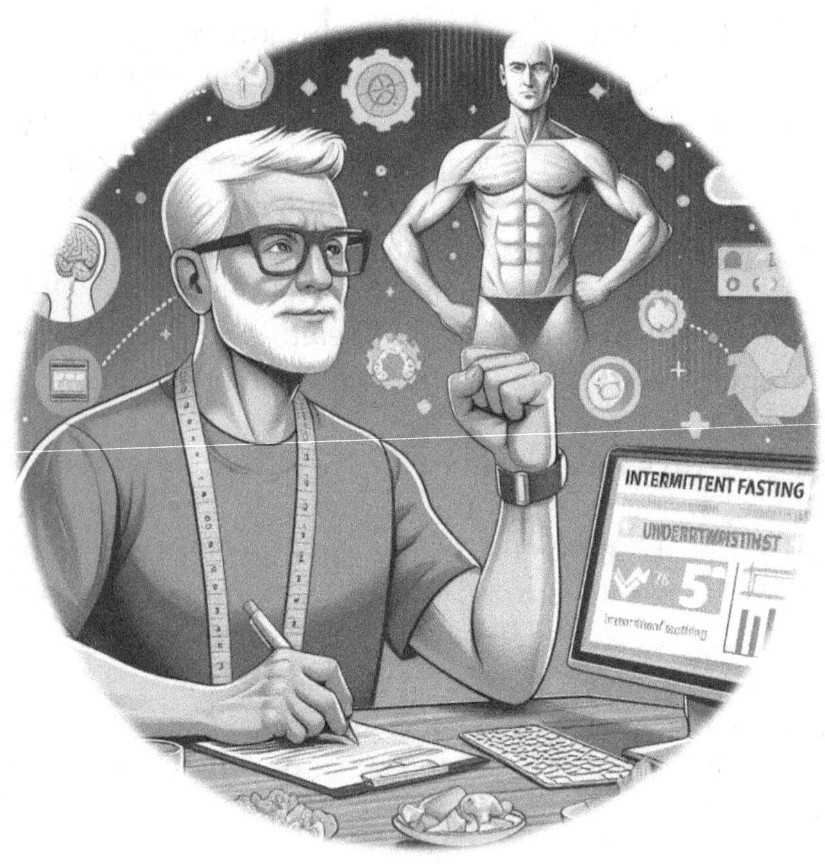

Intermittent fasting (IF) has emerged as a popular and effective approach to health and wellness, particularly for individuals over 50. In this chapter, we'll delve into the fundamentals of intermittent fasting, explore its various forms, examine the scientific evidence supporting its benefits, debunk common myths and misconceptions, address how IF differs for those over 50, and outline the initial steps to embark on your intermittent fasting journey.

Definition and Principles of Intermittent Fasting

At its core, intermittent fasting is not a diet but rather an eating pattern that cycles between periods of fasting and eating. Unlike traditional diets that focus on what you eat, intermittent fasting is more about when you eat. The primary goal is to restrict the window of time during which you consume food, allowing your body to enter a fasting state and reap the associated health benefits.

There are several different approaches to intermittent fasting, each with its own unique fasting and eating windows. However, the underlying principle remains the same: to give your body a break from food intake and allow it to tap into stored energy reserves, leading to various physiological adaptations that promote health and longevity.

Different Types of Intermittent Fasting

One of the appealing aspects of intermittent fasting is its flexibility, as there are several different methods to choose from. Some of the most popular types of intermittent fasting include:

- 16:8 Method: Also known as the Leangains protocol, this approach involves fasting for 16 hours and eating within an 8-hour window each day.
- 5:2 Diet: With this method, you eat normally for five days of the week and restrict your calorie intake to 500-600 calories on two non-consecutive days.
- Alternate-Day Fasting: This approach involves alternating between days of normal eating and days of fasting or significantly reduced calorie intake.
- Eat-Stop-Eat: In this method, you fast for a full 24 hours once or twice a week, consuming no calories during the fasting period.
- Warrior Diet: This approach involves fasting for 20 hours and eating within a 4-hour window each day, typically in the evening.

Each of these methods has its own set of advantages and challenges, so it's essential to choose the approach that aligns best with your lifestyle and goals.

Scientific Evidence Supporting IF

The popularity of intermittent fasting is not merely a result of anecdotal success stories but is also supported by a growing body of scientific research. Studies have shown that intermittent fasting can have numerous benefits for both physical and mental health.

For example, research indicates that intermittent fasting can lead to weight loss, improved metabolic health, reduced inflammation, enhanced cognitive function, and increased longevity. These effects are thought to be mediated by various mechanisms, including changes in hormone levels, increased autophagy (cellular repair), and improved insulin sensitivity.

Moreover, intermittent fasting has been shown to offer protection against chronic diseases such as type 2 diabetes, heart disease, cancer, and neurodegenerative disorders. By promoting metabolic flexibility and reducing oxidative stress, fasting may help prevent and even reverse age-related decline in health.

Common Myths and Misconceptions About IF

Despite its growing popularity, intermittent fasting is still subject to many myths and misconceptions. Some of the most common myths include:

- Fasting leads to muscle loss: Contrary to popular belief, intermittent fasting does not necessarily lead to muscle loss, especially when combined with resistance training.
- Fasting is only for weight loss: While weight loss is a common goal of intermittent fasting, it offers numerous other health benefits beyond just shedding pounds.
- Fasting is unsafe: When done properly, intermittent fasting is generally safe for most people and may even have protective effects on health.
- You must skip breakfast: While some forms of intermittent fasting involve skipping breakfast, it's not a requirement. The key is to find a fasting and eating pattern that works for you.

By debunking these myths and misconceptions, we can better understand the true potential of intermittent fasting and make informed decisions about incorporating it into our lives.

How IF Differs for Individuals Over 50

Intermittent fasting can be particularly beneficial for individuals over 50 due to age-related changes in metabolism, hormone levels, and body composition. As we age, our metabolism slows down, making it more challenging to maintain a healthy weight and prevent age-related diseases.

Moreover, older adults may be more prone to insulin resistance, inflammation, and oxidative stress, all of which can contribute to chronic diseases such as diabetes, heart disease, and Alzheimer's. Intermittent fasting has been shown to address many of these age-related issues by improving metabolic health, reducing inflammation, and promoting cellular repair processes.

However, it's essential to approach intermittent fasting with caution, especially for those with underlying health conditions or taking medications. Consulting with a healthcare professional before starting an intermittent fasting regimen is recommended, particularly for individuals over 50.

Initial Steps to Start Intermittent Fasting

If you're ready to give intermittent fasting a try, here are some initial steps to get started:

- Educate Yourself: Take the time to learn about the different types of intermittent fasting and determine which approach aligns best with your goals and lifestyle.
- Start Slowly: If you're new to fasting, consider easing into it by gradually extending the fasting window over time. Start with a 12-hour fast and gradually increase to 14, 16, or even 18 hours as you become more comfortable.
- Stay Hydrated: Drink plenty of water during your fasting periods to stay hydrated and stave off

hunger.
- Listen to Your Body: Pay attention to how your body responds to fasting and adjust your approach accordingly. If you experience dizziness, weakness, or other adverse effects, consider modifying your fasting regimen or seeking guidance from a healthcare professional.

Be Patient: Rome wasn't built in a day, and neither are the health benefits of intermittent fasting. Give your body time to adapt to the new eating pattern, and don't get discouraged if you don't see immediate results.

By taking these initial steps and approaching intermittent fasting with an open mind and a willingness to experiment, you can unlock the transformative power of this lifestyle approach and reap the numerous benefits it has to offer.

Chapter 02

The Benefits of Intermittent Fasting for the 50+ Population

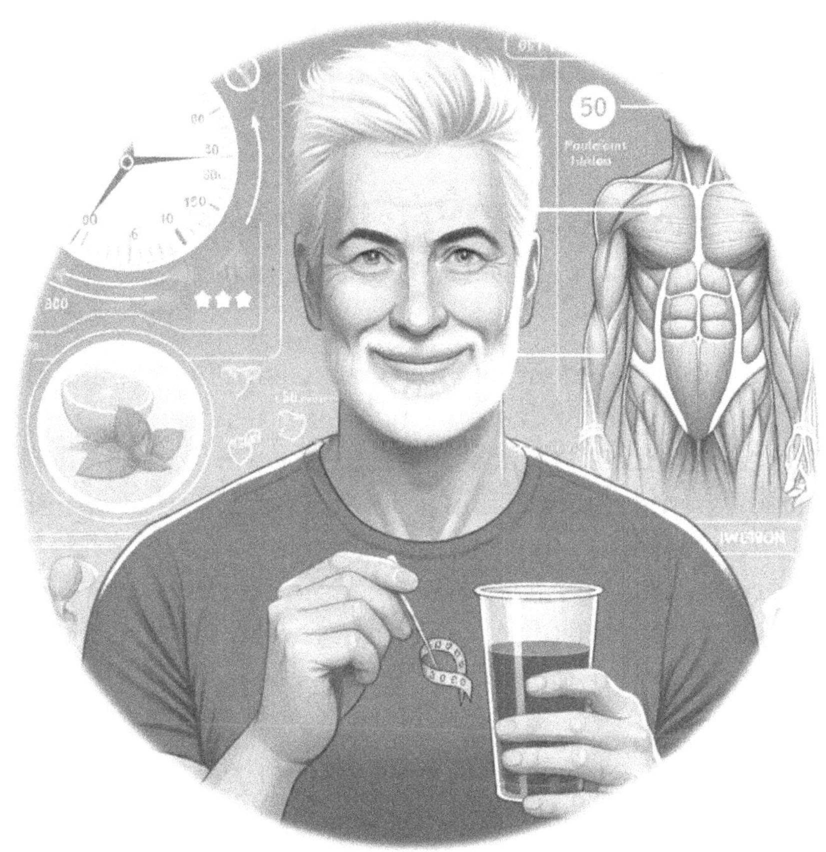

Intermittent fasting (IF) stands as a beacon of hope for individuals over 50, offering a range of benefits that can profoundly impact overall health and well-being. In this chapter, we'll explore how intermittent fasting can enhance weight loss and metabolism, improve cardiovascular health, control blood sugar levels, enhance mental clarity and cognitive function, promote longevity, and provide anti-aging benefits. Additionally, we'll delve deeper into scientific evidence supporting these claims, discuss strategies for successful implementation, and hear testimonials from individuals over 50 who have experienced firsthand the transformative power of intermittent fasting.

Enhanced Weight Loss and Metabolism

Weight management becomes increasingly challenging as we age due to factors such as hormonal changes, decreased muscle mass, and a slower metabolism. Intermittent fasting offers a unique approach to weight loss that extends beyond simple calorie restriction. By incorporating periods of fasting, individuals can optimize fat burning, increase metabolic flexibility, and promote sustainable weight loss.

Aging often brings with it a natural decline in metabolic rate, making it more difficult to maintain a healthy weight. With intermittent fasting, however, individuals can counteract this decline by tapping into stored fat reserves for energy during fasting periods. This shift in fuel utilization promotes ketosis, a metabolic state where the body burns fat for fuel, leading to accelerated fat loss and improved body composition.

Moreover, intermittent fasting has been shown to increase levels of hormones such as norepinephrine and growth hormone, which play critical roles in fat mobilization and metabolism. By harnessing these hormonal changes, individuals can amplify their weight loss efforts and achieve sustainable results.

For individuals over 50 who may struggle with stubborn belly fat or age-related weight gain, intermittent fasting serves as a powerful tool for achieving and maintaining a healthy weight. By adopting a fasting regimen that aligns with their lifestyle and goals, individuals can unlock the transformative potential of intermittent fasting and reclaim control over their health and well-being.

Improved Cardiovascular Health

Heart disease remains a leading cause of morbidity and mortality worldwide, particularly among older adults. Fortunately, intermittent fasting has emerged as a promising strategy for improving cardiovascular health and reducing the risk of heart disease.

Research has consistently demonstrated that

intermittent fasting can lead to improvements in various markers of cardiovascular health, including blood pressure, cholesterol levels, triglycerides, and inflammatory markers. These improvements are thought to be mediated by factors such as reduced oxidative stress, improved insulin sensitivity, and enhanced autophagy (cellular repair).

For example, a study published in the American Journal of Clinical Nutrition found that alternate-day fasting led to significant reductions in LDL cholesterol, triglycerides, and inflammatory markers in overweight and obese adults. Similarly, research published in the journal Obesity Reviews concluded that intermittent fasting can lower blood pressure, improve lipid profiles, and reduce the risk of coronary artery disease.

By promoting cardiovascular health, intermittent fasting can help individuals over 50 reduce their risk of heart disease, stroke, and other cardiovascular conditions, allowing them to enjoy a longer, healthier life. With proper guidance and support, individuals can leverage the cardiovascular benefits of intermittent fasting to optimize their heart health and well-being.

Better Control of Blood Sugar Levels

Type 2 diabetes and insulin resistance are prevalent health concerns among older adults, affecting millions of individuals worldwide. Intermittent fasting offers a promising approach to managing blood sugar levels and improving insulin sensitivity, thereby reducing the risk of developing diabetes and related complications.

Fasting has been shown to lower blood sugar levels, improve insulin sensitivity, and reduce insulin resistance, all of which are critical for maintaining optimal blood glucose control. By allowing the body to rest from constant food intake, intermittent fasting can help regulate blood sugar levels and prevent spikes and crashes throughout the day.

A study published in the journal Cell Metabolism found that time-restricted feeding, a form of intermittent fasting, improved insulin sensitivity, reduced insulin levels, and lowered fasting glucose levels in overweight and obese individuals. Similarly, research published in the journal Obesity Reviews concluded that intermittent fasting can lead to significant improvements in glycemic control and insulin sensitivity, making it an effective strategy for managing diabetes and metabolic syndrome.

For individuals over 50 who may be at increased risk of developing diabetes or struggling to manage their blood sugar levels, intermittent fasting serves as a valuable tool for promoting metabolic health and reducing disease risk. By adopting a fasting regimen that aligns with their needs and preferences, individuals can take control of their diabetes management and improve their overall health and well-being.

Enhanced Mental Clarity and Cognitive Function

Cognitive decline is a common concern as we age, with conditions such as Alzheimer's disease and dementia affecting millions of older adults worldwide. Intermittent fasting offers numerous benefits for brain health, including enhanced mental clarity, improved cognitive function, and protection against age-related neurodegenerative diseases.

Fasting triggers various neuroprotective mechanisms, including increased production of brain-derived neurotrophic factor (BDNF), a protein that supports the growth and survival of neurons. Additionally, fasting promotes the production of ketones, which serve as an alternative fuel source for the brain and have been shown to improve cognitive function and protect against neurodegeneration.

Research published in the journal Neuroscience Letters found that intermittent fasting improved cognitive function and protected against age-related cognitive decline in rats. Similarly, a study published in the journal Molecular and Cellular Neuroscience concluded that intermittent fasting increased hippocampal neurogenesis, a process critical for learning and memory, in mice.

By promoting brain health and cognitive function, intermittent fasting can help individuals over 50 maintain mental sharpness, memory, and overall cognitive vitality as they age. With proper guidance and support, individuals can harness the cognitive benefits of intermittent fasting to optimize their brain health and well-being.

Longevity and Anti-Aging Benefits

One of the most exciting aspects of intermittent fasting is its potential to extend lifespan and promote healthy aging. Studies in animals have consistently shown that calorie restriction and intermittent fasting can increase longevity and delay the onset of age-related diseases.

Fasting triggers various cellular repair processes, including autophagy, which helps remove damaged and dysfunctional components from cells. This promotes cellular health and resilience, reduces the accumulation of age-related damage, and extends lifespan.

Additionally, intermittent fasting has been shown to reduce markers of inflammation and oxidative stress, both of which are implicated in the aging process. By promoting a state of metabolic efficiency and cellular rejuvenation, intermittent fasting can help individuals over 50 not only live longer but also enjoy a higher quality of life in their later years.

A study published in the journal Cell Metabolism found that alternate-day fasting extended lifespan and improved healthspan in mice, leading to reductions in age-related diseases such as cancer, cardiovascular disease, and neurodegenerative disorders. Similarly, research published in the journal Nature Communications concluded that intermittent fasting increased lifespan and delayed age-related decline in C. elegans, a model organism used in aging research.

By promoting longevity and anti-aging benefits, intermittent fasting offers individuals over 50 the opportunity to age gracefully and maintain their health and vitality well into their later years. With proper guidance and support, individuals can leverage the longevity benefits of intermittent fasting to optimize their healthspan and enjoy a longer, healthier life.

Scientific Evidence Supporting IF

The benefits of intermittent fasting are not merely anecdotal but are supported by a robust body of scientific research. Numerous studies have demonstrated the efficacy of intermittent fasting for weight loss, metabolic health, cardiovascular function, cognitive function, and longevity.

For example, a systematic review and meta-analysis published in the journal Obesity Reviews found that intermittent fasting led to significant reductions in body weight, body fat percentage, and waist circumference in overweight and obese individuals. Similarly, a review article published in the journal Cell Metabolism concluded that intermittent fasting can improve metabolic health, reduce inflammation, and extend lifespan in various organisms, including humans.

Moreover, a study published in the New England Journal of Medicine found that alternate-day fasting led to significant improvements in cardiovascular risk factors such as LDL cholesterol, triglycerides, and blood pressure. Similarly, research published in the journal Diabetes Care concluded that intermittent fasting improved glycemic control, insulin sensitivity, and beta-cell function in individuals with type 2 diabetes.

By synthesizing findings from diverse areas of research, scientists have established a compelling case for the benefits of intermittent fasting across the lifespan. From weight management and metabolic health to cardiovascular function and cognitive function, intermittent fasting offers a multifaceted approach to promoting health and well-being in individuals over 50.

Testimonials from Individuals Over 50

To illustrate the real-world impact of intermittent fasting on the 50+ population, let's hear from individuals who have experienced firsthand the transformative power of this lifestyle approach:

- **Testimonial 1:** "As someone in my late 50s, I struggled with weight gain and low energy for years. After starting intermittent fasting, I've lost over 30 pounds, gained muscle, and feel more energetic than ever. Not only has fasting helped me shed excess weight, but it's also improved my overall health and vitality."

- **Testimonial 2:** "Intermittent fasting has been a game-changer for my cardiovascular health. As someone with high blood pressure and cholesterol, I was worried about my risk of heart disease. Since starting fasting, my blood pressure has dropped, my cholesterol levels have improved, and I feel more confident about my heart health moving forward."

- **Testimonial 3:** "I never realized how much of an impact intermittent fasting could have on my mental clarity and cognitive function. As someone in my 60s, I was starting to notice subtle changes in my memory and focus. But after incorporating fasting into my routine, I feel sharper, more alert, and better able to handle mental tasks. It's like a fog has lifted, and I feel like myself again."

These testimonials highlight the diverse ways in which intermittent fasting can benefit individuals over 50, from weight loss and cardiovascular health to cognitive function and overall well-being. By sharing their stories, these individuals inspire others to embrace intermittent fasting and unlock the transformative potential it holds for promoting health and vitality in the 50+ population.

Conclusion

As we've explored in this chapter, intermittent fasting offers a wealth of benefits for individuals over 50, ranging from enhanced weight loss and metabolic health to improved cardiovascular function, better blood sugar control, sharper cognitive function, and increased longevity. Supported by scientific evidence and real-world testimonials, intermittent fasting emerges as a powerful tool for promoting health, vitality, and longevity in the 50+ population.

By adopting a fasting regimen that aligns with their needs and preferences, individuals over 50 can harness the transformative power of intermittent fasting and reclaim control over their health and well-being. With proper guidance and support, they can navigate the challenges and uncertainties of aging with confidence, knowing that they have a powerful ally in their corner: intermittent fasting.

As we continue our journey into the world of intermittent fasting, let's embrace the opportunity to optimize our health, extend our vitality, and live our best lives, no matter our age. With intermittent fasting as our guide, we can embark on a path of lifelong health and well-being, empowered to thrive at every stage of life.

Chapter 03

The Science Behind Intermittent Fasting

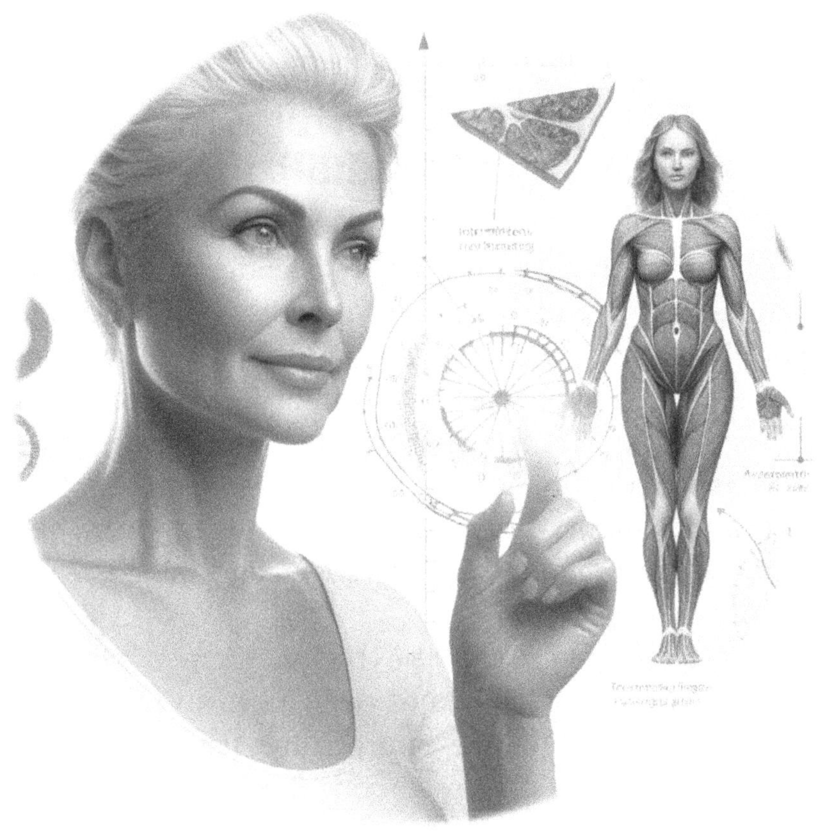

Intermittent fasting (IF) isn't just a trend; it's a scientifically grounded approach to health and wellness. In this chapter, we'll delve into the intricate mechanisms through which intermittent fasting affects the body's metabolism, the role of hormones like insulin, the cellular repair processes triggered by fasting, its impact on inflammation and oxidative stress, scientific studies relevant to the 50+ age group, and the body's adaptation to intermittent fasting over time.

How Intermittent Fasting Affects the Body's Metabolism

Intermittent fasting induces a cascade of metabolic changes that optimize energy utilization and promote overall health. When we fast, our bodies transition from using glucose as the primary fuel source to utilizing stored fat for energy. This shift is facilitated by reduced insulin levels and increased secretion of counter-regulatory hormones such as glucagon, which stimulate the breakdown of glycogen and fat stores.

During fasting periods, the body enters a state of ketosis, where ketone bodies derived from fatty acids serve as alternative fuel sources for tissues like the brain and muscles. This metabolic flexibility allows the body to adapt to periods of nutrient scarcity and maintain energy balance over time.

Moreover, intermittent fasting enhances mitochondrial function and biogenesis, leading to improved energy production and efficiency. By promoting mitochondrial health, intermittent fasting may help mitigate age-related declines in metabolic function and support overall vitality and well-being.

The Role of Insulin and Other Hormones in IF

Insulin plays a central role in regulating energy metabolism and nutrient partitioning in the body. When we eat, insulin levels rise, signaling cells to take up glucose from the bloodstream and store it as glycogen or fat for later use. In contrast, during fasting periods, insulin levels decrease, allowing the body to access stored energy reserves and maintain blood glucose levels within a narrow range.

Intermittent fasting helps restore insulin sensitivity and reduce insulin resistance, particularly in individuals with metabolic disorders like type 2 diabetes. By promoting a more balanced and responsive insulin signaling pathway, intermittent fasting can help improve glucose control, reduce the risk of insulin resistance, and prevent the development of diabetes and related complications.

Additionally, intermittent fasting modulates the secretion of other hormones such as growth hormone, which plays a role in fat metabolism, muscle growth, and tissue repair. By optimizing hormonal balance, intermittent fasting supports metabolic health and promotes overall well-being.

Cellular Repair Processes Triggered by Fasting

One of the key mechanisms through which intermittent fasting exerts its health benefits is by triggering cellular repair processes such as autophagy and apoptosis. Autophagy is a cellular recycling process in which damaged or dysfunctional components are broken down and recycled to generate new cellular material. This helps clear out accumulated debris and maintain cellular health and function.

During fasting periods, the body upregulates autophagy as a means of conserving energy and promoting cellular repair and regeneration. By clearing out damaged proteins and organelles, autophagy helps maintain cellular homeostasis and protects against age-related decline.

Moreover, intermittent fasting stimulates apoptosis, or programmed cell death, in damaged or senescent cells. This helps remove potentially harmful cells from the body and prevents them from proliferating and causing further damage.

Together, these cellular repair processes promote tissue renewal, enhance resilience to stress, and support overall longevity and well-being.

Impact on Inflammation and Oxidative Stress

Chronic inflammation and oxidative stress are implicated in the pathogenesis of numerous age-related diseases, including cardiovascular disease, cancer, and neurodegenerative disorders. Intermittent fasting exerts anti-inflammatory and antioxidant effects that help mitigate these processes and promote overall health.

Studies have shown that intermittent fasting can reduce levels of pro-inflammatory cytokines and markers of oxidative stress, thereby lowering systemic inflammation and oxidative damage. By modulating immune function and oxidative pathways, intermittent fasting helps maintain a balanced inflammatory response and protect against chronic disease.

Moreover, intermittent fasting enhances the body's stress response mechanisms, including the production of heat shock proteins and other molecular chaperones. These proteins help protect cells from stress-induced damage and promote cellular resilience and longevity.

Scientific Studies and Findings Relevant to the 50+ Age Group

Numerous studies have investigated the effects of intermittent fasting on health outcomes in individuals over 50, yielding promising results. For example, a study published in the journal JAMA Internal Medicine found that alternate-day fasting improved cardiovascular risk factors such as blood pressure, LDL cholesterol, and triglycerides in overweight and obese adults aged 50-69 years.

Similarly, research published in the journal Cell Metabolism demonstrated that time-restricted feeding improved insulin sensitivity, reduced liver fat, and increased fat oxidation in older adults with prediabetes. These findings suggest that intermittent fasting may offer significant benefits for metabolic health and disease prevention in individuals over 50.

Moreover, a study published in the journal Neurobiology of Aging found that intermittent fasting improved cognitive function and reduced markers of neuroinflammation and oxidative stress in aged mice. These findings support the potential neuroprotective effects of intermittent fasting and its relevance for promoting brain health in older adults.

The Body's Adaptation to Intermittent Fasting Over Time

As individuals continue to practice intermittent fasting, their bodies undergo various adaptations that optimize metabolic efficiency and promote overall health. For example, over time, individuals may experience increased fat oxidation, improved insulin sensitivity, and enhanced mitochondrial function, leading to greater energy production and vitality.

Moreover, intermittent fasting may lead to changes in gene expression and epigenetic regulation that support long-term health and longevity. By modulating gene pathways related to metabolism, inflammation, and stress resistance, intermittent fasting helps maintain cellular homeostasis and protect against age-related decline.

Additionally, individuals may notice improvements in appetite regulation, food cravings, and eating behavior as they become accustomed to fasting periods. By promoting mindful eating and a greater awareness of hunger and satiety cues, intermittent fasting fosters a healthier relationship with food and eating.

Conclusion

In conclusion, intermittent fasting is grounded in solid scientific principles that underpin its numerous health benefits. By modulating metabolism, hormone levels, cellular repair processes, inflammation, and oxidative stress, intermittent fasting promotes overall health and well-being in individuals over 50.

Through a deeper understanding of the science behind intermittent fasting, individuals can harness its transformative potential to optimize their healthspan and enjoy a longer, healthier life. With proper guidance and support, intermittent fasting can serve as a powerful tool for promoting metabolic health, cognitive function, cardiovascular wellness, and longevity in the 50+ age group.

As we continue our exploration of intermittent fasting, let's embrace the opportunity to unlock the secrets of optimal health and vitality, one fast at a time. By integrating intermittent fasting into our lives, we can embark on a journey of lifelong wellness and well-being, empowered to thrive at every stage of life.

Chapter 04

Getting Started with Intermittent Fasting

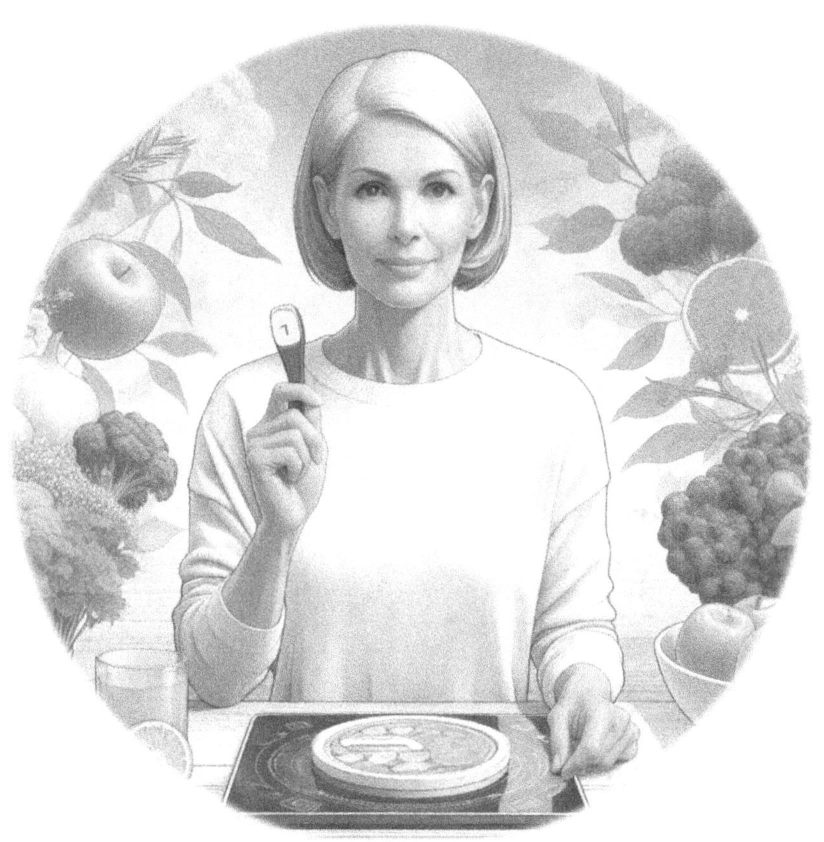

Embarking on the journey of intermittent fasting can be both exciting and daunting. This chapter is dedicated to guiding you through the process of getting started with intermittent fasting effectively. We'll cover essential steps such as assessing your current health status, consulting with healthcare professionals, setting realistic goals and expectations, choosing the right type of fasting for you, implementing gradual strategies, tracking progress, and staying motivated. By following these steps, you'll be equipped to begin your intermittent fasting journey with confidence and determination.

Assessing Your Current Health Status

Before diving into intermittent fasting, it's crucial to assess your current health status comprehensively. Start by evaluating factors such as your medical history, existing health conditions, medications you're taking, and your overall lifestyle habits. Consider scheduling a visit with your healthcare provider to discuss your interest in intermittent fasting and to address any concerns you may have regarding its suitability for your health.

During your assessment, pay attention to key health metrics such as blood pressure, blood glucose levels, cholesterol levels, and body composition. These measurements can provide valuable insights into your current health status and serve as baseline markers for tracking progress over time. Additionally, consider factors such as stress levels, sleep quality, physical activity levels, and nutritional intake, as these can influence your ability to adhere to an intermittent fasting regimen.

By conducting a thorough assessment of your health status, you can identify any potential risk factors or contraindications that may impact your ability to fast safely. This knowledge will enable you to make informed decisions about incorporating intermittent fasting into your lifestyle and to tailor your fasting approach to suit your individual needs and circumstances.

Consulting with Healthcare Professionals

Seeking guidance from healthcare professionals is essential when embarking on an intermittent fasting journey, particularly if you have underlying health conditions or are taking medications. Schedule an appointment with your primary care physician, registered dietitian, or other qualified healthcare provider to discuss your interest in intermittent fasting and to receive personalized recommendations based on your unique health profile.

During your consultation, be sure to share relevant information about your medical history, current health status, medications, and lifestyle habits. Your healthcare provider can help you assess the potential risks and benefits of intermittent fasting in the context of your individual health needs and goals. They can also provide guidance on how to implement intermittent fasting safely and effectively, taking into account any medical considerations or dietary restrictions you may have.

Additionally, consider consulting with other healthcare professionals such as a registered dietitian or nutritionist who specializes in intermittent fasting. These professionals can offer personalized dietary recommendations, meal planning assistance, and ongoing support to help you navigate the challenges of fasting and optimize your nutritional intake during feeding periods.

By collaborating with healthcare professionals, you can gain valuable insights into how intermittent fasting may impact your health and receive tailored guidance to support your fasting journey effectively.

Setting Realistic Goals and Expectations

Setting realistic goals is essential for success with intermittent fasting. Take the time to identify your specific health objectives and establish clear, achievable goals that align with your aspirations and lifestyle. Whether your goal is to lose weight, improve metabolic health, enhance energy levels, or simply optimize overall well-being, ensure that it is specific, measurable, attainable, relevant, and time-bound (SMART).

When setting goals for intermittent fasting, consider factors such as your current health status, medical history, lifestyle habits, and personal preferences. Be realistic about what you hope to achieve and the timeframe in which you expect to see results. Remember that intermittent fasting is not a quick fix or a one-size-fits-all solution, and it may take time to experience meaningful changes in your health and well-being.

Once you've established your goals, break them down into smaller, actionable steps that you can work towards gradually. Celebrate your progress along the way and acknowledge the effort you're putting into improving your health and lifestyle. By setting realistic goals and expectations, you'll set yourself up for success and maintain motivation throughout your intermittent fasting journey.

Choosing the Right Type of Fasting for You

One of the most critical decisions you'll make when starting intermittent fasting is choosing the fasting method that best suits your needs, preferences, and lifestyle. There are several different approaches to intermittent fasting, each with its unique fasting and eating patterns. Experiment with different fasting protocols to find the one that feels most sustainable and effective for you.

Some common intermittent fasting methods include:

- **16:8 Method:** This approach involves fasting for 16 hours each day and restricting eating to an 8-hour window, typically from noon to 8 p.m. or 1 p.m. to 9 p.m.

- **5:2 Diet:** With this method, you eat normally for five days of the week and restrict calorie intake to 500-600 calories on two non-consecutive days.

- **Alternate-Day Fasting:** This approach involves alternating between days of normal eating and days of fasting or significantly reduced calorie intake.

- **Eat-Stop-Eat:** With this method, you fast for a full 24 hours once or twice a week, consuming no calories during the fasting period.

- **Warrior Diet:** This approach involves fasting for 20 hours each day and eating within a 4-hour window, typically in the evening.

Consider factors such as your schedule, daily routine, hunger levels, and dietary preferences when choosing a fasting method. Start with a method that feels manageable and gradually experiment with different approaches to find what works best for you. Remember that there is no one-size-fits-all approach to intermittent fasting, and it may take time to discover the fasting regimen that aligns with your goals and lifestyle.

Implementing Gradual Strategies

For individuals new to intermittent fasting, it's essential to implement gradual strategies to ease into the fasting regimen and allow your body time to adjust. Begin by gradually extending the fasting window over several days or weeks, starting with a shorter fasting duration and gradually increasing the fasting period as you become more comfortable.

For example, start by fasting for 12 hours overnight and gradually extend the fasting window by an hour each day until you reach your desired fasting duration. Alternatively, experiment with intermittent fasting on non-consecutive days to allow your body time to rest and recover between fasting periods.

During fasting periods, focus on staying hydrated and consuming nutrient-dense foods during eating windows to support overall health and well-being. Pay attention to your body's hunger and satiety cues and adjust your fasting approach as needed to ensure that it aligns with your goals and preferences.

Be patient with yourself as you navigate the challenges of intermittent fasting and remember that it's normal to experience some discomfort or adjustment period initially. Listen to your body, practice self-compassion, and prioritize your health and well-being above all else.

Tracking Progress and Staying Motivated

Tracking your progress is essential for staying motivated and accountable on your intermittent fasting journey. Keep a journal or use a smartphone app to log your fasting and eating times, as well as any changes in weight, body composition, energy levels, and overall well-being.

Celebrate small victories and milestones along the way, such as reaching your fasting goals, noticing improvements in energy levels, or achieving weight loss milestones. Use visual cues such as progress photos or measurements to track changes in body composition over time and stay motivated to continue your journey.

Additionally, seek support from friends, family, or online communities who share similar goals and experiences. Surround yourself with positive influences and seek encouragement from others who have successfully implemented intermittent fasting into their lives.

By tracking your progress and staying motivated, you can stay committed to your intermittent fasting journey and reap the numerous benefits it has to offer. Remember that intermittent fasting is a lifestyle change, and it may take time to see significant results.

Stay consistent, stay focused, and trust the process as you work towards achieving your health and wellness goals.

Conclusion

Getting started with intermittent fasting requires careful planning, preparation, and commitment. By assessing your current health status, consulting with healthcare professionals, setting realistic goals and expectations, choosing the right fasting method, implementing gradual strategies, tracking progress, and staying motivated, you can embark on your intermittent fasting journey with confidence and determination.

Remember that intermittent fasting is not a one-size-fits-all approach, and it may take time to find the fasting regimen that works best for you. Be patient with yourself, listen to your body, and stay focused on your health goals. With dedication and perseverance, intermittent fasting can become a sustainable and rewarding lifestyle habit that supports your health, vitality, and well-being for years to come.

Embrace the journey, stay positive, and enjoy the transformative benefits of intermittent fasting on your path to optimal health and wellness. With the right mindset and support system in place, you can achieve your health and wellness goals and unlock your full potential with intermittent fasting.

Chapter 05

Customizing Your Fasting Plan

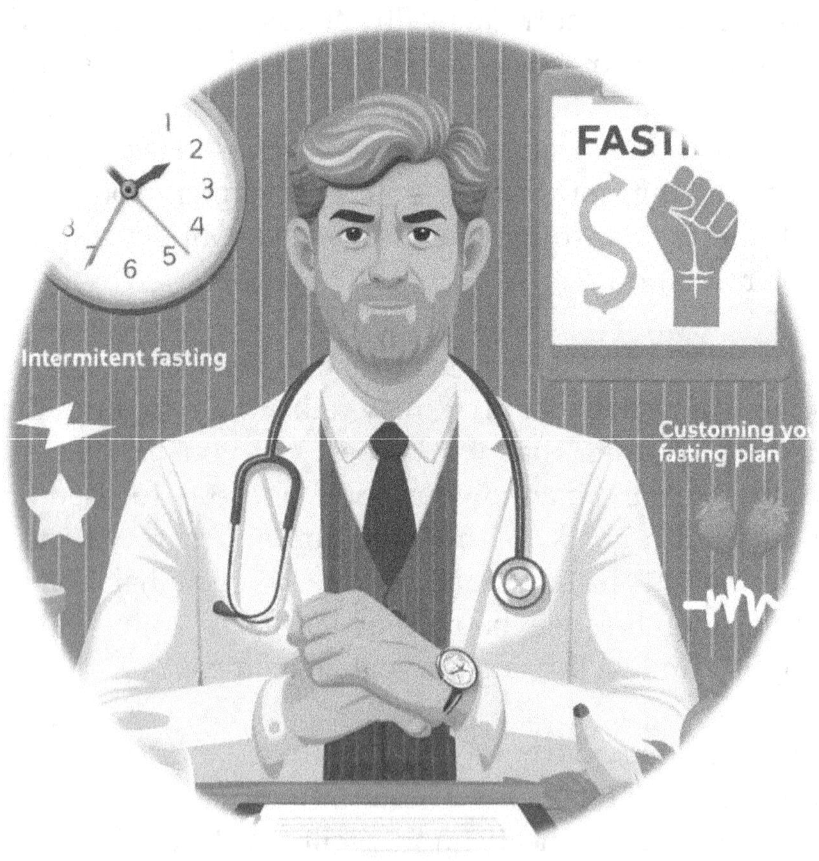

Intermittent fasting is not a one-size-fits-all approach. In this chapter, we'll explore how to customize your fasting plan to suit your unique needs, preferences, and lifestyle. From identifying your individual requirements to adjusting fasting windows, incorporating physical activity, managing social situations, tailoring your plan for specific health conditions, and providing examples of personalized fasting plans, you'll learn how to make intermittent fasting work for you.

Identifying Your Unique Needs and Preferences

The first step in customizing your fasting plan is to identify your unique needs and preferences. Consider factors such as your schedule, daily routine, hunger levels, energy requirements, dietary preferences, and health goals. Reflect on what motivates you to pursue intermittent fasting and what obstacles you may encounter along the way.

Ask yourself questions such as:

- When do I feel most hungry or least hungry during the day?
- What times of day do I have the most energy for physical activity or exercise?
- Are there certain foods or beverages I prefer to consume during fasting and eating windows?
- Do I have any dietary restrictions or health conditions that may impact my fasting plan?

By gaining clarity on your individual requirements and preferences, you can tailor your fasting plan to suit your lifestyle and optimize your chances of success.

Adjusting Fasting Windows to Fit Your Lifestyle

One of the key advantages of intermittent fasting is its flexibility. Experiment with different fasting windows to find the schedule that aligns best with your lifestyle and preferences. Some common fasting protocols include:

- 16:8 Method: Fasting for 16 hours each day and eating within an 8-hour window.
- 5:2 Diet: Eating normally for five days of the week and restricting calorie intake on two non-consecutive days.
- Alternate-Day Fasting: Alternating between days of normal eating and days of fasting or significantly reduced calorie intake.
- Eat-Stop-Eat: Fasting for a full 24 hours once or twice a week.
- Warrior Diet: Fasting for 20 hours each day and eating within a 4-hour window.

Experiment with different fasting protocols to determine which one feels most sustainable and effective for you. Consider factors such as your work schedule, social commitments, exercise routine, and meal preferences when selecting a fasting schedule. Remember that intermittent fasting is meant to enhance your quality of life, so choose a fasting plan that fits seamlessly into your daily routine.

Incorporating Physical Activity and Exercise

Physical activity and exercise are essential components of a healthy lifestyle, and they can complement your intermittent fasting regimen effectively. Determine the best time to incorporate physical activity into your fasting schedule based on your energy levels, workout preferences, and daily routine.

Some individuals prefer to exercise in a fasted state, while others find it more comfortable to work out during their eating window. Experiment with different approaches to see what works best for you and enhances your performance and recovery. Listen to your body and adjust your exercise routine as needed to accommodate your fasting schedule.

Remember to stay hydrated and fuel your body with nutritious foods to support your energy levels and recovery from exercise. Incorporating a combination of cardiovascular exercise, strength training, flexibility, and mobility work can help you achieve optimal health and fitness while fasting.

Managing Social Situations and Dining Out

Social situations and dining out can present challenges when following an intermittent fasting regimen, but with some planning and preparation, you can navigate these scenarios successfully. Communicate your fasting goals and preferences with friends, family, and dining companions to enlist their support and understanding.

When dining out, choose restaurants that offer options that align with your fasting plan, such as salads, lean protein, vegetables, and whole grains. Be mindful of portion sizes and avoid excessive consumption of high-calorie, high-fat foods that may derail your progress. If necessary, modify menu items to fit your dietary preferences and restrictions.

Consider bringing a snack or meal with you when attending social events or gatherings to ensure that you have suitable options available. Plan ahead and communicate with hosts or organizers to accommodate your dietary needs whenever possible.

Tailoring Your Plan for Specific Health Conditions

If you have specific health conditions or dietary restrictions, it's essential to tailor your fasting plan accordingly to ensure that it supports your overall health and well-being. Consult with healthcare professionals, such as your primary care physician or a registered dietitian, to receive personalized recommendations based on your individual needs and circumstances.

Individuals with conditions such as diabetes, hypertension, cardiovascular disease, gastrointestinal disorders, or eating disorders may require modifications to their fasting plan to accommodate their health needs safely. Your healthcare provider can help you develop a fasting plan that aligns with your health goals and minimizes potential risks.

Consider factors such as medication timing, blood sugar management, hydration, and nutritional requirements when customizing your fasting plan for specific health conditions. Be proactive in monitoring your health and seek professional guidance if you experience any adverse effects or concerns while fasting.

Examples of Personalized Fasting Plans

To illustrate how intermittent fasting can be customized to suit individual needs and preferences, let's explore a few examples of personalized fasting plans:

Example 1: Busy Professional

- Fasting Protocol: 16:8 Method
- Fasting Schedule: Fast from 8 p.m. to 12 p.m. (16-hour fast)
- Eating Window: Eat from 12 p.m. to 8 p.m.
- Lifestyle Considerations: Schedule workouts in the morning before breaking the fast. Plan meals and snacks in advance to avoid impulse eating during the fasting period.

Example 2: Stay-at-Home Parent

- Fasting Protocol: Alternate-Day Fasting
- Fasting Schedule: Fast on Mondays, Wednesdays, and Fridays
- Eating Window: Eat normally on Tuesdays, Thursdays, Saturdays, and Sundays
- Lifestyle Considerations: Use fasting days to focus on self-care activities, rest, and relaxation. Plan family meals and activities on non-fasting days to maintain social connections and enjoyment.

Example 3: Fitness Enthusiast

- Fasting Protocol: Eat-Stop-Eat
- Fasting Schedule: Fast for 24 hours once or twice a week (e.g., Mondays and Thursdays)
- Eating Window: Eat normally on non-fasting days
- Lifestyle Considerations: Schedule intense workouts on non-fasting days to optimize performance and recovery. Plan meals to include adequate protein, carbohydrates, and fats to support muscle growth and repair.

These examples demonstrate how intermittent fasting can be customized to accommodate diverse lifestyles, preferences, and health goals effectively. Experiment with different fasting protocols, meal timings, and lifestyle adjustments to find the approach that works best for you.

Conclusion

Customizing your fasting plan is essential for optimizing the effectiveness and sustainability of intermittent fasting. By identifying your unique needs and preferences, adjusting fasting windows to fit your lifestyle, incorporating physical activity and exercise, managing social situations and dining out, tailoring your plan for specific health conditions, and exploring examples of personalized fasting plans, you can develop a fasting regimen that supports your overall health and well-being.

Remember that intermittent fasting is a flexible and adaptable approach to health and wellness. Be open to experimentation, listen to your body, and make adjustments as needed to ensure that your fasting plan aligns with your goals and preferences. With dedication, patience, and perseverance, intermittent fasting can become a valuable tool for optimizing your health, vitality, and longevity for years to come.

Embrace the journey of self-discovery and empowerment as you explore the transformative benefits of intermittent fasting on your path to optimal health and well-being. With the right approach and mindset, you can harness the power of intermittent fasting to unlock your full potential and live your best life.

Chapter 06

Nutrition and Intermittent Fasting

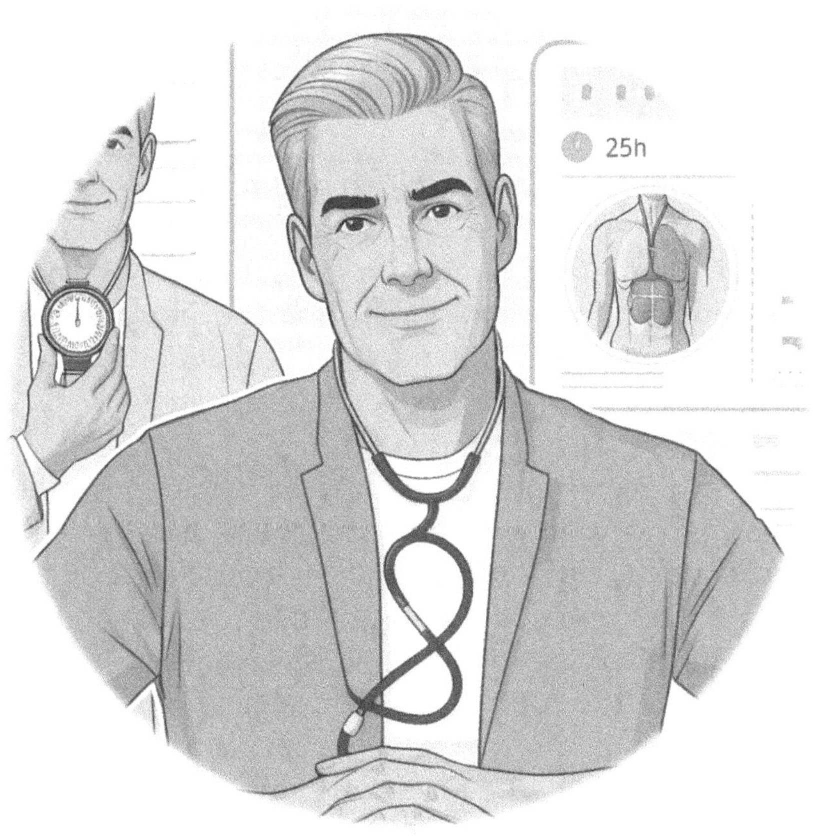

In this chapter, we'll delve into the crucial role of nutrition in supporting your intermittent fasting journey. From the importance of nutrient-dense foods to recommended options for breaking your fast, avoiding common dietary pitfalls, understanding the role of hydration, supplement recommendations, and sample balanced meal ideas, you'll gain insights into how to nourish your body effectively while practicing intermittent fasting.

Importance of Nutrient-Dense Foods

Nutrition plays a pivotal role in optimizing health and well-being, especially during periods of fasting. When following an intermittent fasting regimen, it's essential to prioritize nutrient-dense foods that provide essential vitamins, minerals, antioxidants, and macronutrients to support overall health and vitality.

Focus on incorporating a variety of whole foods into your diet, including fruits, vegetables, lean proteins, whole grains, nuts, seeds, and legumes. These foods are rich in essential nutrients and fiber, which can help promote satiety, regulate blood sugar levels, support digestive health, and reduce the risk of chronic disease.

Limit your intake of processed foods, refined sugars, unhealthy fats, and artificial additives, which offer little nutritional value and may contribute to inflammation, insulin resistance, and weight gain. By prioritizing nutrient-dense foods, you can nourish your body effectively and enhance the benefits of intermittent fasting.

Recommended Foods for Breaking Your Fast

Breaking your fast mindfully is essential for maintaining stable blood sugar levels, replenishing energy stores, and supporting overall well-being. When ending a fasting period, opt for nutrient-rich, easily digestible foods that provide sustained energy and promote satiety.

Some recommended options for breaking your fast include:

- Protein-rich foods: Incorporate lean protein sources such as poultry, fish, eggs, tofu, tempeh, and legumes to support muscle repair and growth.
- Complex carbohydrates: Choose whole grains like quinoa, brown rice, oats, and sweet potatoes to provide sustained energy and fiber for digestive health.
- Healthy fats: Include sources of healthy fats such as avocados, nuts, seeds, olive oil, and fatty fish to promote satiety and support brain health.
- Fruits and vegetables: Incorporate a variety of colorful fruits and vegetables to provide essential vitamins, minerals, antioxidants, and hydration.

Avoid consuming large quantities of high-sugar, high-fat, or processed foods immediately after fasting, as this can lead to rapid spikes in blood sugar levels and potential digestive discomfort. Instead, opt for balanced, nutrient-rich meals that support your overall health and well-being.

Avoiding Common Dietary Pitfalls

While intermittent fasting can offer numerous health benefits, it's essential to be mindful of common dietary pitfalls that may undermine your progress. Avoid falling into the trap of unhealthy eating habits, such as:

- Overcompensating for fasting periods by consuming excessive calories or indulging in unhealthy foods.
- Relying on processed snacks, sugary beverages, or convenience foods to break your fast quickly.
- Neglecting proper hydration or failing to replenish electrolytes during fasting periods.
- Skipping meals or depriving yourself of essential nutrients needed for optimal health.

Be mindful of your dietary choices and strive to maintain balance, moderation, and variety in your eating patterns. Focus on nourishing your body with whole, nutrient-dense foods that support your health goals and promote long-term well-being.

Hydration and Its Role in Fasting

Proper hydration is essential for supporting overall health and well-being, especially during periods of fasting. Drinking an adequate amount of water helps regulate body temperature, support digestion, transport nutrients, flush out toxins, and maintain electrolyte balance.

During fasting periods, it's essential to prioritize hydration and drink water regularly to prevent dehydration and support optimal bodily function. Aim to consume at least 8-10 glasses of water per day, or more if you're physically active or live in a hot climate.

In addition to water, you can also incorporate other hydrating beverages such as herbal teas, infused water, coconut water, and electrolyte-rich drinks to replenish fluids and electrolytes lost during fasting. Avoid excessive consumption of caffeinated or sugary beverages, as these can contribute to dehydration and disrupt your fasting regimen.

Supplement Recommendations

While intermittent fasting can provide numerous health benefits, it's essential to ensure that you're meeting your nutritional needs adequately. Consider incorporating certain supplements into your routine to address potential nutrient deficiencies and support overall health and well-being.

Some recommended supplements for individuals practicing intermittent fasting include:

- Multivitamin: Choose a high-quality multivitamin

to provide essential vitamins and minerals that may be lacking in your diet due to restricted eating windows.

- Omega-3 fatty acids: Consider supplementing with fish oil or algae-based omega-3 supplements to support cardiovascular health, brain function, and inflammation.
- Vitamin D: Opt for a vitamin D supplement to maintain optimal levels of this essential nutrient, especially if you have limited sun exposure or live in northern latitudes.
- Electrolytes: Consider supplementing with electrolyte tablets or powders to replenish sodium, potassium, magnesium, and other essential electrolytes lost during fasting periods.
- Probiotics: Support gut health and digestion by incorporating a high-quality probiotic supplement containing beneficial bacteria.

Before starting any new supplements, consult with a healthcare professional or registered dietitian to ensure they are safe and appropriate for your individual needs and health status.

Sample Balanced Meal Ideas

To help you get started with incorporating nutrient-dense foods into your intermittent fasting regimen, here are some sample balanced meal ideas:

Breakfast:

- Scrambled eggs with spinach, mushrooms, and bell peppers
- Whole grain toast with avocado and sliced tomatoes

Greek yogurt parfait with mixed berries and almonds

Lunch:

Grilled chicken salad with mixed greens, cherry tomatoes, cucumbers, and balsamic vinaigrette

- Quinoa and black bean bowl with roasted vegetables and salsa
- Lentil soup with whole grain bread and a side of steamed broccoli

Dinner:

- Baked salmon with quinoa pilaf and roasted Brussels sprouts
- Stir-fried tofu with broccoli, bell peppers, and brown rice
- Turkey chili with kidney beans, diced tomatoes, onions, and spices

Snacks:

- Apple slices with almond butter
- Greek yogurt with honey and walnuts
- Hummus and vegetable crudites

These sample meal ideas provide a balanced combination of protein, carbohydrates, healthy fats, fiber, vitamins, and minerals to support your nutritional needs while practicing intermittent fasting. Experiment with different ingredients and flavors to create meals that suit your taste preferences and dietary requirements.

Conclusion

Nutrition plays a vital role in supporting your overall health and well-being, especially during periods of intermittent fasting. By prioritizing nutrient-dense foods, breaking your fast mindfully, avoiding common dietary pitfalls, staying hydrated, incorporating appropriate supplements, and exploring sample balanced meal ideas, you can nourish your body effectively and optimize the benefits of intermittent fasting.

Remember to listen to your body, practice moderation, and strive for balance in your eating patterns. By making informed dietary choices and prioritizing your nutritional needs, you can enhance the effectiveness and sustainability of your intermittent fasting regimen and support your long-term health and well-being.

Embrace the opportunity to explore new flavors, ingredients, and meal combinations as you embark on your journey towards optimal health and vitality with intermittent fasting. With the right approach to nutrition, you can fuel your body for success and enjoy the transformative benefits of intermittent fasting for years to come.

Chapter 07

Overcoming Common Challenges

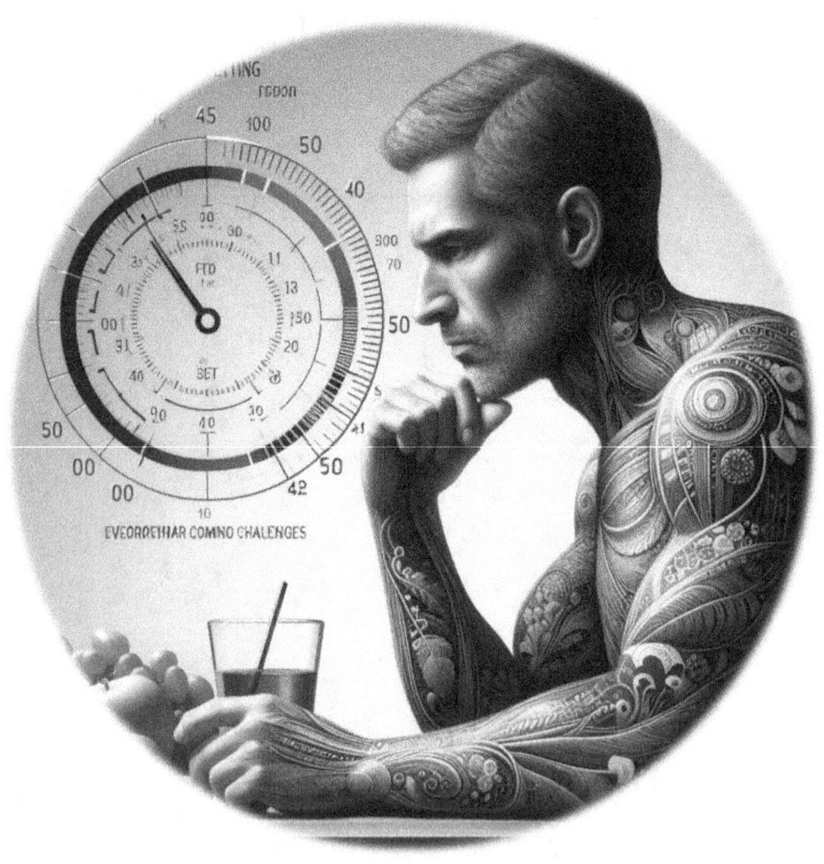

Embarking on an intermittent fasting journey can bring about various challenges that may test your resolve and commitment. In this chapter, we'll explore strategies for overcoming common hurdles encountered while practicing intermittent fasting. From dealing with hunger and cravings to managing energy levels, coping with social dynamics, handling setbacks and plateaus, staying committed, and accessing resources and support systems, you'll learn how to navigate obstacles effectively and sustain your fasting practice for long-term success.

Dealing with Hunger and Cravings

Hunger and cravings are common experiences, especially when adjusting to a new eating pattern like intermittent fasting. To manage hunger and cravings effectively, try the following strategies:

- Stay hydrated: Drinking water can help suppress appetite and keep you feeling full between meals. Aim to drink at least 8-10 glasses of water per day, or more if you're physically active.
- Choose filling foods: Prioritize nutrient-dense, high-fiber foods that promote satiety and help you feel satisfied for longer periods. Incorporate protein-rich foods, healthy fats, and complex carbohydrates into your meals to keep hunger at bay.
- Practice mindful eating: Pay attention to hunger and satiety cues, and eat slowly and mindfully to fully enjoy your meals. Avoid distractions such as

TV or smartphones while eating to prevent mindless overeating.

- Plan meals and snacks: Prepare nutritious meals and snacks in advance to avoid impulsive food choices or reaching for unhealthy options when hunger strikes. Having healthy options readily available can help you stay on track with your fasting goals.

Managing Energy Levels and Fatigue

During the initial stages of intermittent fasting, you may experience fluctuations in energy levels and periods of fatigue as your body adjusts to the new eating pattern. To manage energy levels and combat fatigue, try the following strategies:

- Prioritize sleep: Aim for 7-9 hours of quality sleep each night to support energy levels, cognitive function, and overall well-being. Establish a consistent sleep schedule and create a relaxing bedtime routine to promote restful sleep.
- Fuel your body appropriately: Consume balanced meals and snacks that provide a combination of protein, carbohydrates, and healthy fats to sustain energy levels throughout the day. Avoid skipping meals or restricting calories excessively, as this can lead to fatigue and lethargy.
- Incorporate regular physical activity: Engage in regular exercise or physical activity to boost energy levels, improve mood, and reduce feelings of fatigue. Choose activities you enjoy and aim for at

least 30 minutes of moderate-intensity exercise most days of the week.

- Take breaks and rest: Listen to your body and take breaks when needed to rest and recharge. Incorporate relaxation techniques such as deep breathing, meditation, or gentle stretching to reduce stress and promote relaxation.

Coping with Social and Family Dynamics

Navigating social and family dynamics while practicing intermittent fasting can present unique challenges, especially during social gatherings or family meals. To cope with social situations effectively, consider the following strategies:

- Communicate openly: Share your fasting goals and preferences with friends, family, and loved ones to enlist their support and understanding. Explain how intermittent fasting works and why it's important to you, and encourage open dialogue about your dietary choices.
- Plan ahead: Anticipate social events or gatherings where food may be present and plan your fasting and eating schedule accordingly. Consider adjusting your fasting window or meal timing to accommodate social commitments while staying true to your fasting goals.
- Focus on socializing: Shift the focus of social gatherings away from food and towards meaningful connections with others. Engage in

activities such as conversation, games, or outdoor adventures that don't revolve around eating.

- Bring your own food: If attending a gathering where food options may be limited or not aligned with your dietary preferences, consider bringing a dish or snack that fits your fasting plan. This allows you to enjoy the event while staying true to your nutritional goals.

Handling Setbacks and Plateaus

Setbacks and plateaus are a natural part of any health and wellness journey, including intermittent fasting. Instead of becoming discouraged, use setbacks and plateaus as opportunities for growth and learning. Try the following strategies for overcoming setbacks and plateaus:

- Reflect on the root cause: Identify the factors contributing to the setback or plateau, such as changes in lifestyle, stress, lack of consistency, or external triggers. Reflect on what you can learn from the experience and how you can adjust your approach moving forward.
- Reassess your goals: Take a step back and revisit your goals and motivations for practicing intermittent fasting. Are they still relevant and meaningful to you? Consider adjusting your goals or setting new milestones to keep yourself motivated and focused.
- Seek support: Reach out to friends, family, or online communities for support and

encouragement during challenging times. Share your experiences, ask for advice, and lean on others for guidance and reassurance.

- Stay consistent: Consistency is key to overcoming setbacks and breaking through plateaus. Stick to your fasting schedule, prioritize healthy eating habits, and remain committed to your long-term health and wellness goals. Trust the process and stay patient as you work towards achieving your desired outcomes.

Strategies for Staying Committed

Staying committed to your intermittent fasting practice requires dedication, discipline, and perseverance, especially when faced with obstacles or temptations. To maintain your commitment to fasting, try the following strategies:

- Set clear intentions: Clarify your reasons for practicing intermittent fasting and define your goals and expectations. Write down your intentions and review them regularly to stay focused and motivated.
- Establish a routine: Create a consistent fasting and eating schedule that aligns with your daily routine and preferences. Establishing a routine can help you develop habits and rituals that support your fasting practice and make it easier to stick to over time.
- Find accountability partners: Surround yourself with supportive individuals who share similar

goals and experiences with intermittent fasting. Partner with a friend, family member, or online buddy to hold each other accountable, celebrate successes, and provide encouragement during challenging times.

- Practice self-care: Prioritize self-care activities that nourish your body, mind, and spirit. Make time for relaxation, stress management, and activities you enjoy to maintain a healthy balance and prevent burnout.

- Stay adaptable: Remain flexible and open-minded as you navigate your intermittent fasting journey. Be willing to adjust your approach, experiment with different strategies, and learn from your experiences to find what works best for you.

Resources and Support Systems

Accessing resources and support systems can be instrumental in sustaining your intermittent fasting practice and overcoming challenges along the way. Consider the following resources and support systems to enhance your fasting journey:

- Books and articles: Explore books, articles, and online resources that provide information and guidance on intermittent fasting, nutrition, and healthy lifestyle habits. Look for evidence-based sources written by reputable experts in the field.

- Apps and technology: Utilize smartphone apps, fitness trackers, or online platforms designed to support intermittent fasting and track your progress. These tools can help you monitor fasting and eating windows, log meals, and stay motivated with reminders and notifications.

- Online communities: Join online forums, social media groups, or virtual communities dedicated to intermittent fasting and healthy living. Engage with like-minded individuals, share experiences, ask questions, and seek support from peers who understand your journey.

- Professional guidance: Consider seeking guidance from healthcare professionals, such as registered dietitians, nutritionists, or fasting experts, who can provide personalized recommendations and support based on your individual needs and goals. A qualified professional can offer tailored advice, address specific concerns, and help you navigate challenges effectively.

Conclusion

Overcoming common challenges encountered while practicing intermittent fasting requires resilience, determination, and a willingness to adapt. By implementing strategies to manage hunger and cravings, regulate energy levels, navigate social dynamics, overcome setbacks and plateaus, stay committed, and access resources and support systems, you can sustain your fasting practice and reap the numerous health benefits it offers.

Remember that intermittent fasting is a journey, not a destination, and it's normal to encounter obstacles along the way. Approach challenges with a growth mindset, embrace opportunities for learning and growth, and celebrate your progress and achievements as you work towards achieving your health and wellness goals with intermittent fasting.

With patience, perseverance, and support, you can overcome any challenge that comes your way and emerge stronger, healthier, and more resilient than ever before. Embrace the journey, stay committed to your goals, and trust in your ability to thrive with intermittent fasting for a lifetime of health and vitality.

Chapter 08

Intermittent Fasting and Exercise

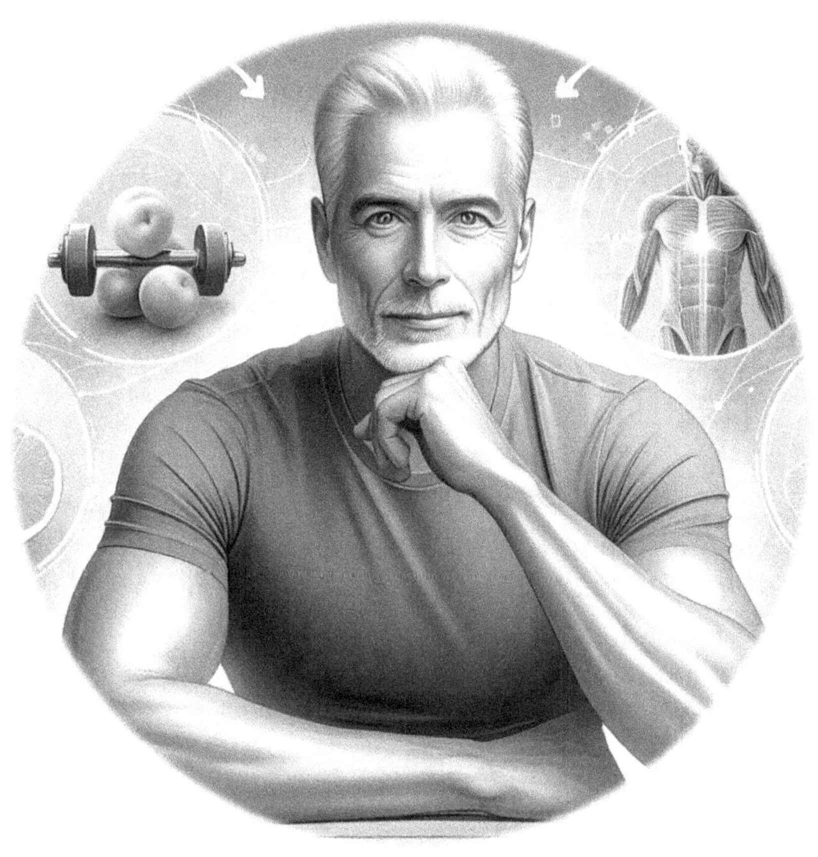

Integrating exercise into your intermittent fasting routine can amplify the benefits of both practices, promoting overall health, fitness, and well-being. In this chapter, we'll explore the advantages of combining intermittent fasting with exercise, the best types of exercises for individuals over 50, strategies for timing workouts with fasting windows, adjusting intensity and duration of workouts, prioritizing recovery and injury prevention, and providing sample exercise routines to support your fitness goals.

Benefits of Combining IF with Exercise

Combining intermittent fasting with regular exercise can synergistically enhance numerous aspects of health and fitness, including:

- Weight management: Intermittent fasting and exercise work together to promote fat loss, preserve lean muscle mass, and improve body composition.
- Metabolic health: Both practices can enhance insulin sensitivity, regulate blood sugar levels, and support metabolic function.
- Cardiovascular health: Exercise and intermittent fasting have been shown to improve cardiovascular health markers such as blood pressure, cholesterol levels, and heart rate variability.
- Muscle strength and endurance: Regular exercise, particularly resistance training, can increase

muscle strength and endurance, while intermittent fasting may promote muscle protein synthesis and optimize muscle recovery.

- Brain health: Exercise and intermittent fasting have neuroprotective effects, supporting cognitive function, memory, and mood regulation.
- Longevity: Both practices have been linked to longevity and may promote cellular repair, reduce inflammation, and enhance stress resistance.

By combining intermittent fasting with exercise, you can maximize the benefits of both practices and support your overall health and well-being effectively.

Best Types of Exercises for Individuals Over 50

When incorporating exercise into your intermittent fasting routine, it's essential to choose activities that are safe, effective, and enjoyable, especially as you age. Some of the best types of exercises for individuals over 50 include:

- Strength training: Resistance training using free weights, machines, resistance bands, or bodyweight exercises can help maintain muscle mass, improve bone density, and support functional independence.
- Cardiovascular exercise: Aerobic activities such as walking, cycling, swimming, or dancing can improve cardiovascular health, endurance, and circulation.

- Flexibility and mobility work: Stretching exercises, yoga, tai chi, or Pilates can enhance flexibility, mobility, balance, and coordination, reducing the risk of falls and injuries.
- Low-impact activities: Low-impact exercises such as walking, elliptical training, or water aerobics are gentle on the joints and suitable for individuals with arthritis, joint pain, or mobility issues.

Choose activities that align with your fitness level, preferences, and goals, and consult with a healthcare professional or fitness expert if you have any underlying health concerns or medical conditions.

Timing Workouts with Fasting Windows

The timing of your workouts relative to your fasting windows can influence your energy levels, performance, and recovery. Consider the following strategies for timing workouts effectively:

- Fasted workouts: Some individuals prefer to exercise in a fasted state, typically in the morning before breaking their fast. Fasted workouts may enhance fat burning and metabolic adaptations, but it's essential to listen to your body and ensure you have adequate energy and hydration.
- Fed workouts: Others may prefer to exercise during or shortly after their eating window when they have consumed nutrients and energy. Eating a balanced meal or snack containing carbohydrates,

protein, and healthy fats before a workout can provide fuel for exercise and support muscle repair and recovery.

- Experimentation: Experiment with different timing strategies to determine what works best for you. Pay attention to how your body responds to exercise in a fasted versus fed state and adjust your approach accordingly.

Ultimately, the best time to work out is when you feel most energized, focused, and motivated, whether that's during a fasting window or after eating.

Adjusting Intensity and Duration of Workouts

As you age, it's essential to adjust the intensity and duration of your workouts to accommodate changes in fitness level, recovery capacity, and injury risk. Consider the following guidelines for adjusting exercise intensity and duration:

- Start gradually: Begin with low to moderate-intensity exercise and gradually increase intensity, duration, and frequency over time as your fitness improves.
- Listen to your body: Pay attention to how your body responds to exercise and adjust the intensity or duration as needed to prevent fatigue, discomfort, or injury. Focus on quality over quantity and prioritize proper form and technique.
- Incorporate variety: Include a variety of exercises

and activities in your workout routine to target different muscle groups, prevent boredom, and reduce the risk of overuse injuries. Incorporate strength training, cardiovascular exercise, flexibility work, and balance training for a well-rounded fitness program.

- Rest and recovery: Allow adequate time for rest and recovery between workouts to prevent overtraining and promote muscle repair and adaptation. Incorporate active recovery days, foam rolling, stretching, and other recovery modalities to support recovery and reduce muscle soreness.

By adjusting the intensity and duration of your workouts to match your current fitness level and recovery capacity, you can maintain a safe and effective exercise routine while practicing intermittent fasting.

Recovery and Injury Prevention

Prioritizing recovery and injury prevention is essential for maintaining long-term health and fitness, especially as you age. Consider the following strategies for supporting recovery and reducing the risk of injury:

- Prioritize sleep: Aim for 7-9 hours of quality sleep each night to support muscle repair, hormone regulation, and overall recovery. Create a relaxing bedtime routine, optimize your sleep environment, and prioritize consistency in your sleep schedule.

- Fuel your body: Consume balanced meals and snacks containing carbohydrates, protein, and healthy fats to replenish energy stores, support muscle repair, and enhance recovery. Choose nutrient-dense foods that provide essential vitamins, minerals, and antioxidants to support overall health and well-being.
- Hydrate properly: Stay hydrated before, during, and after exercise to maintain fluid balance, regulate body temperature, and support cellular function. Drink water regularly throughout the day and consider consuming electrolyte-rich beverages during prolonged or intense workouts.
- Incorporate rest days: Allow adequate time for rest and recovery between workouts to prevent overtraining and reduce the risk of injury. Schedule regular rest days or active recovery days to give your body time to recover and rejuvenate.
- Listen to your body: Pay attention to signs of fatigue, soreness, or discomfort, and adjust your exercise routine as needed to prevent overuse injuries or burnout. Be mindful of any changes in performance, mobility, or pain and consult with a healthcare professional if you experience persistent or severe symptoms.

By prioritizing recovery and injury prevention, you can maintain a balanced and sustainable exercise routine that supports your health and fitness goals over the long term.

Sample Exercise Routines

To help you get started with incorporating exercise into your intermittent fasting routine, here are some sample exercise routines tailored for individuals over 50:

Strength Training Routine:

- Warm-up: 5-10 minutes of light cardio or dynamic stretching
- Strength exercises: Perform 8-12 repetitions of each exercise, focusing on major muscle groups such as legs, chest, back, shoulders, and arms. Choose compound exercises such as squats, lunges, chest presses, rows, shoulder presses, and biceps curls.
- Cool-down: 5-10 minutes of stretching to improve flexibility and reduce muscle tension

Cardiovascular Exercise Routine:

- Warm-up: 5-10 minutes of brisk walking, cycling, or low-impact cardio
- Cardiovascular exercise: Choose an activity you enjoy such as walking, cycling, swimming, or dancing and aim for 20-30 minutes of moderate-intensity exercise. Gradually increase intensity or duration as fitness improves.
- Cool-down: 5-10 minutes of gentle stretching to promote flexibility and relaxation

Flexibility and Mobility Routine:

- Warm-up: 5-10 minutes of dynamic stretching or foam rolling
- Flexibility exercises: Perform a series of static stretches targeting major muscle groups, focusing on areas of tightness or restriction. Include stretches for the hamstrings, quadriceps, calves, hips, chest, shoulders, and back.
- Mobility exercises: Incorporate dynamic mobility drills to improve joint range of motion, stability, and coordination. Include exercises such as leg swings, arm circles, hip circles, and spinal rotations.

Experiment with different exercise routines, modalities, and intensities to find what works best for you and fits your schedule, preferences, and fitness goals.

Conclusion

Integrating exercise into your intermittent fasting routine can enhance the benefits of both practices, promoting overall health, fitness, and well-being. By combining intermittent fasting with regular exercise, you can support weight management, metabolic health, cardiovascular function, muscle strength and endurance, brain health, and longevity effectively.

Choose exercises that are safe, enjoyable, and suitable for your fitness level and preferences, and prioritize proper nutrition, hydration, recovery, and injury prevention to support your exercise routine. Experiment with different timing strategies, adjust the intensity and duration of your workouts, and listen to your body to optimize your exercise experience while practicing intermittent fasting.

With a balanced and sustainable approach to exercise and intermittent fasting, you can achieve your health and fitness goals and enjoy a vibrant and active lifestyle for years to come. Embrace the opportunity to move your body, challenge yourself, and experience the transformative benefits of exercise and intermittent fasting on your journey to optimal health and well-being.

Chapter 09

Mental and Emotional Well-being

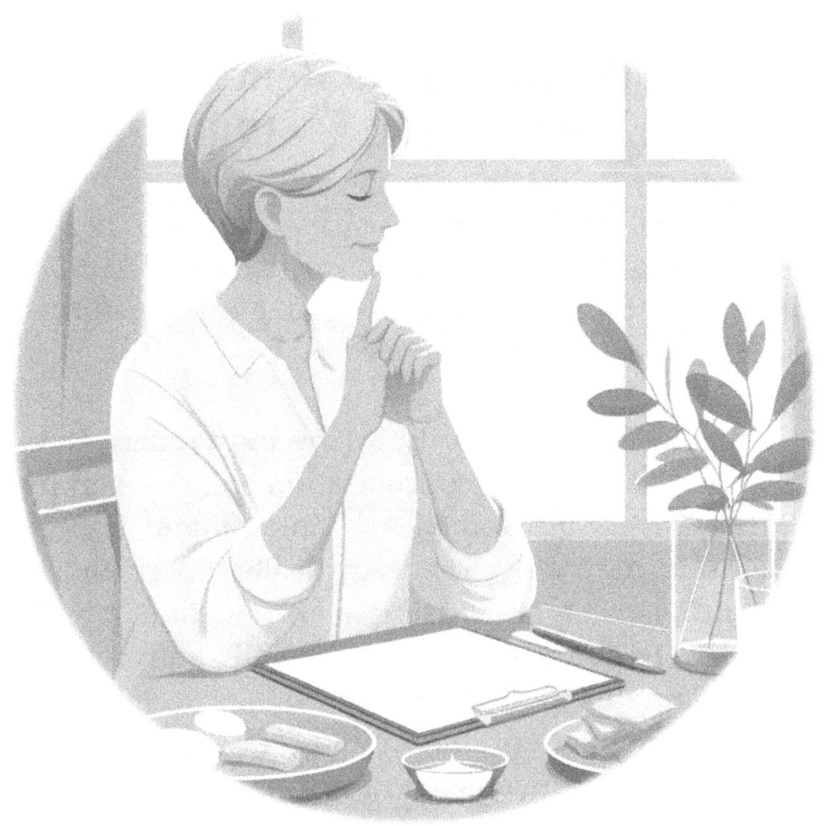

In this chapter, we'll explore the profound impact of intermittent fasting on mental and emotional well-being. From the psychological benefits of intermittent fasting to strategies for managing stress, emotional eating, cultivating mindfulness, building a positive relationship with food, setting and achieving mental health goals, and sharing personal stories and experiences, you'll discover how intermittent fasting can contribute to a healthier mind and spirit.

The Psychological Benefits of Intermittent Fasting

Intermittent fasting extends its benefits beyond physical health to encompass mental and emotional well-being. Some of the psychological benefits of intermittent fasting include:

- Enhanced mental clarity: Many individuals report improved focus, concentration, and cognitive function while practicing intermittent fasting. Fasting may enhance brain health by promoting neuroplasticity, increasing the production of brain-derived neurotrophic factor (BDNF), and reducing inflammation in the brain.
- Mood regulation: Intermittent fasting has been linked to improvements in mood, stress resilience, and emotional well-being. Fasting may stimulate the release of feel-good neurotransmitters such as serotonin and dopamine, which can promote feelings of happiness and well-being.
- Stress reduction: Fasting may have stress-reducing

effects on the body, helping to regulate the stress response, lower cortisol levels, and promote relaxation. By supporting stress resilience, intermittent fasting may improve overall mental health and resilience to adversity.

By incorporating intermittent fasting into your lifestyle, you may experience a range of psychological benefits that contribute to a greater sense of well-being and vitality.

Managing Stress and Emotional Eating

Stress and emotional eating can undermine your efforts to practice intermittent fasting and achieve your health goals. To manage stress and emotional eating effectively, consider the following strategies:

- Identify triggers: Pay attention to the situations, emotions, or thoughts that trigger stress or emotional eating. Common triggers may include boredom, loneliness, anxiety, sadness, or social pressure. By identifying your triggers, you can develop strategies to address them more effectively.
- Practice stress management techniques: Incorporate stress management techniques into your daily routine to reduce tension, promote relaxation, and support emotional well-being. Techniques such as deep breathing, progressive muscle relaxation, mindfulness meditation, yoga, or journaling can help you cope with stress in a

healthy way.

- Find alternative coping strategies: Instead of turning to food for comfort or distraction, explore alternative coping strategies to manage stress and emotions. Engage in activities you enjoy, such as reading, listening to music, spending time outdoors, or connecting with friends and loved ones. Find healthy ways to soothe yourself and nurture your emotional well-being.
- Address underlying issues: If stress or emotional eating persists despite your efforts to manage it, consider seeking support from a mental health professional or counselor. Therapy can provide valuable tools and strategies for addressing underlying issues, developing coping skills, and promoting emotional resilience.

By taking proactive steps to manage stress and emotional eating, you can cultivate a healthier relationship with food and support your overall well-being while practicing intermittent fasting.

Mindfulness and Meditation Practices

Mindfulness and meditation practices can complement intermittent fasting by promoting present-moment awareness, reducing stress, and supporting emotional balance. Consider incorporating the following mindfulness techniques into your daily routine:

- Mindful eating: Practice mindful eating by paying attention to the sensory experience of eating, such

as the taste, texture, aroma, and appearance of food. Slow down, chew your food thoroughly, and savor each bite. Notice the sensations of hunger and fullness without judgment.
- Meditation: Set aside time each day for meditation practice to quiet the mind, cultivate inner peace, and enhance self-awareness. Find a quiet space, sit comfortably, and focus on your breath or a specific mantra or visualization. Allow thoughts and emotions to arise without attachment, gently returning your focus to the present moment.
- Body scan: Conduct a body scan meditation to bring awareness to different areas of your body and release tension or discomfort. Start at the top of your head and systematically scan down through your body, noticing any sensations or areas of tension. Breathe into each area and allow it to relax and soften.

By incorporating mindfulness and meditation practices into your intermittent fasting routine, you can cultivate greater self-awareness, resilience, and emotional well-being.

Building a Positive Relationship with Food

Developing a positive relationship with food is essential for supporting your overall health and well-being, especially while practicing intermittent fasting. Consider the following strategies for building a healthy relationship with food:

- Practice intuitive eating: Listen to your body's hunger and fullness cues and honor your cravings and preferences without judgment. Eat when you're hungry and stop when you're satisfied, paying attention to how different foods make you feel.
- Focus on nourishment: Shift your focus from restrictive dieting or calorie counting to nourishing your body with nutrient-dense, whole foods that support your health and well-being. Choose foods that provide essential vitamins, minerals, antioxidants, and macronutrients to fuel your body effectively.
- Enjoy all foods in moderation: Adopt a balanced approach to eating that allows for flexibility and enjoyment. Instead of labeling foods as "good" or "bad," strive for moderation and variety in your diet. Allow yourself to indulge in occasional treats or favorite foods without guilt or shame.
- Cultivate gratitude: Practice gratitude for the food you have access to and the nourishment it provides for your body and soul. Take time to appreciate the flavors, textures, and aromas of your meals, and savor each bite with mindfulness and gratitude.

By fostering a positive relationship with food based on mindfulness, self-compassion, and nourishment, you can support your overall health and well-being while practicing intermittent fasting.

Setting and Achieving Mental Health Goals

Setting and achieving mental health goals can empower you to cultivate resilience, well-being, and fulfillment in your life. Consider the following steps for setting and achieving mental health goals:

- Reflect on your values and priorities: Take time to reflect on what matters most to you in life and identify areas of your mental health and well-being that you'd like to improve. Consider your values, passions, strengths, and areas for growth.
- Set SMART goals: Create specific, measurable, achievable, relevant, and time-bound (SMART) goals that align with your values and priorities. Break larger goals into smaller, actionable steps that you can work towards consistently over time.
- Create a plan of action: Develop a plan of action outlining the steps you'll take to achieve your mental health goals. Identify potential obstacles or challenges and brainstorm strategies for overcoming them. Set realistic timelines and milestones to track your progress.
- Stay accountable: Hold yourself accountable for your mental health goals by regularly reviewing your progress, celebrating successes, and adjusting your approach as needed. Share your goals with supportive friends, family members, or a therapist who can provide encouragement, feedback, and accountability.
- Practice self-care: Prioritize self-care activities that

support your mental health and well-being, such as getting enough sleep, engaging in regular exercise, practicing relaxation techniques, spending time in nature, and nurturing meaningful relationships.

- Seek support when needed: Don't hesitate to seek support from a mental health professional or counselor if you're struggling with mental health challenges or need guidance and support in achieving your goals. Therapy can provide valuable tools, insights, and resources for overcoming obstacles and creating positive change.

By setting and achieving mental health goals that align with your values and priorities, you can enhance your overall well-being and cultivate a life of purpose, fulfillment, and resilience.

Personal Stories and Experiences

Personal stories and experiences can provide valuable insights, inspiration, and encouragement for others on their journey to improved mental and emotional well-being with intermittent fasting. Consider sharing your own experiences, challenges, and successes with intermittent fasting and how it has impacted your mental and emotional health. By sharing your story, you can connect with others, offer support and encouragement, and foster a sense of community and belonging.

In conclusion, intermittent fasting offers a holistic

approach to promoting mental and emotional well-being, complementing physical health benefits with psychological and emotional advantages. By practicing mindfulness, managing stress and emotional eating, cultivating a positive relationship with food, setting and achieving mental health goals, and sharing personal stories and experiences, you can harness the transformative power of intermittent fasting to nourish your mind, body, and spirit for a life of vitality and well-being.

Chapter 10

Monitoring Your Progress

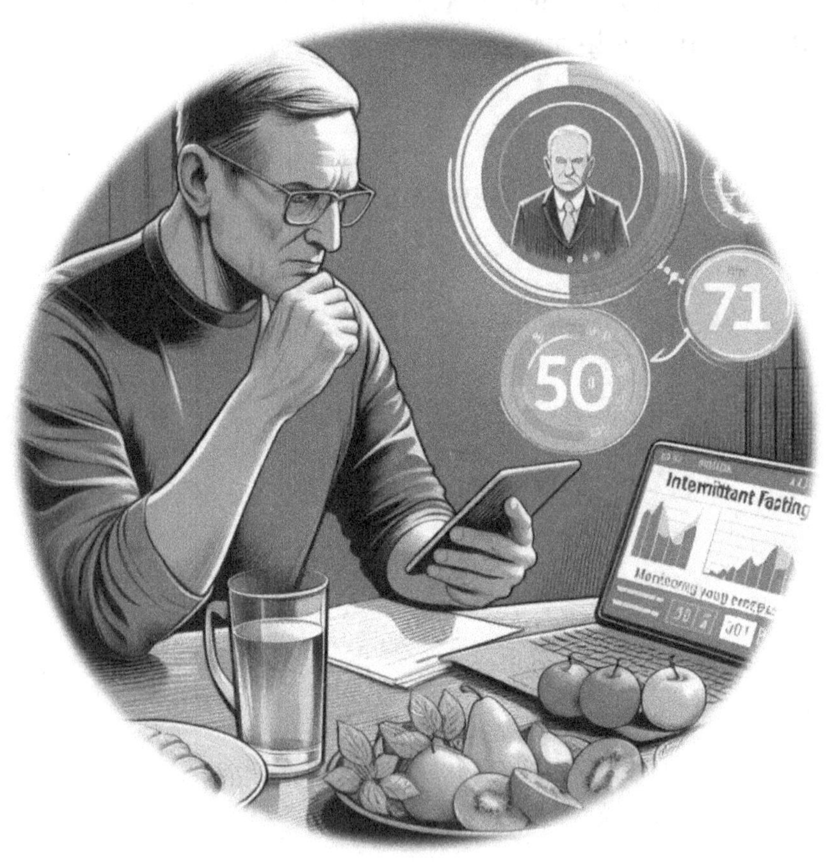

Tracking your progress is essential for staying on course, adjusting your approach as needed, and celebrating your achievements along the way. In this chapter, we'll explore key metrics to track, utilizing journals and apps for tracking, the importance of regular health check-ups and assessments, adjusting your plan based on progress, celebrating milestones and achievements, and implementing long-term maintenance strategies to sustain your success with intermittent fasting.

Key Metrics to Track

Monitoring key metrics allows you to gauge your progress, identify areas for improvement, and stay motivated on your intermittent fasting journey. Some key metrics to track include:

- Weight: Regularly weigh yourself using a reliable scale to track changes in body weight over time. Keep in mind that weight fluctuations can occur due to factors such as hydration status, food intake, and hormonal changes.
- Measurements: Take measurements of key areas such as waist circumference, hips, chest, arms, and thighs to track changes in body composition and inches lost.
- Body fat percentage: Use methods such as body fat scales, calipers, or bioelectrical impedance analysis (BIA) to measure body fat percentage and assess changes in lean muscle mass and fat mass.

- Energy levels: Pay attention to changes in your energy levels, mood, and overall well-being throughout the day. Note any improvements in energy, mental clarity, and physical performance.

- Hunger and satiety: Keep a log of your hunger and satiety levels before, during, and after fasting periods to assess how well your body adapts to intermittent fasting.

- Physical performance: Track improvements in physical performance metrics such as strength, endurance, flexibility, and mobility through exercise and activity.

By monitoring these key metrics regularly, you can track your progress, identify trends, and make informed decisions about your intermittent fasting plan.

Using Journals and Apps for Tracking

Journals and apps can be valuable tools for tracking your progress, recording your experiences, and staying organized with your intermittent fasting journey. Consider using the following methods for tracking:

- Paper journal: Keep a dedicated journal or notebook where you can record your daily fasting and eating times, meals, snacks, physical activity, mood, energy levels, and any observations or reflections. Use the journal to track your progress over time and identify patterns or trends.

- Mobile apps: Explore mobile apps designed specifically for tracking intermittent fasting, such as fasting timers, meal trackers, calorie counters, and habit trackers. These apps often provide features such as reminders, progress charts, and community support to help you stay accountable and motivated.

- Online tools: Utilize online tools and resources, such as spreadsheets, calculators, or tracking templates, to monitor key metrics and track progress toward your goals. Customize these tools to suit your preferences and goals, and update them regularly with new data.

Whether you prefer the simplicity of a paper journal or the convenience of a mobile app, find a tracking method that works best for you and supports your intermittent fasting journey effectively.

Regular Health Check-ups and Assessments

In addition to self-monitoring, regular health check-ups and assessments are essential for ensuring your well-being and detecting any potential health issues. Schedule regular appointments with healthcare professionals, such as your primary care physician, registered dietitian, or fasting specialist, to monitor the following:

- Physical health: Undergo routine physical exams, blood tests, and screenings to assess your overall health, including blood pressure, cholesterol levels, blood sugar levels, and other key markers of health.

- Nutritional status: Consult with a registered dietitian or nutritionist to assess your nutritional status, dietary intake, and nutrient needs. Address any deficiencies or imbalances through dietary modifications or supplementation.

- Metabolic health: Monitor changes in metabolic health markers such as insulin sensitivity, inflammation, and oxidative stress, which may be influenced by intermittent fasting and lifestyle factors.

- Mental and emotional well-being: Discuss any changes in mood, stress, or mental health symptoms with a mental health professional or counselor. Address any concerns or challenges related to stress management, emotional well-being, or psychological health.

By prioritizing regular health check-ups and assessments, you can proactively manage your health and well-being and address any issues that arise in a timely manner.

Adjusting Your Plan Based on Progress

As you progress with intermittent fasting, you may need to adjust your plan based on changes in your goals, preferences, and results. Consider the following factors when making adjustments:

- Progress towards goals: Evaluate your progress towards your health and wellness goals, such as weight loss, muscle gain, improved metabolic health, or increased energy levels. Adjust your fasting protocol, meal timing, or calorie intake as needed to support your goals.

- Adaptation: Pay attention to how your body responds to intermittent fasting over time. If you experience changes in hunger, energy levels, or physical performance, consider modifying your fasting schedule, meal composition, or exercise routine to better align with your body's needs.

- Plateaus or setbacks: If you encounter plateaus or setbacks in your progress, reassess your approach and identify potential areas for improvement. Experiment with different fasting protocols, meal patterns, or lifestyle factors to overcome obstacles and break through barriers.

- Feedback from healthcare professionals: Seek feedback and guidance from healthcare professionals, such as your primary care physician, registered dietitian, or fasting specialist, when making adjustments to your plan. Consider their recommendations and expertise in tailoring your intermittent fasting approach to support your health and well-being effectively.

By staying flexible and responsive to changes in your body and progress, you can optimize your intermittent fasting plan for long-term success and sustainability.

Celebrating Milestones and Achievements

Celebrating milestones and achievements along your intermittent fasting journey is essential for staying motivated, reinforcing positive habits, and acknowledging your progress. Consider the following ways to celebrate your successes:

- Set milestones: Break down your long-term goals into smaller, achievable milestones that you can celebrate along the way. Whether it's reaching a certain weight, fitting into a smaller clothing size, or achieving a personal best in a fitness goal, celebrate each milestone as a sign of progress and accomplishment.

- Reward yourself: Treat yourself to rewards or incentives for reaching milestones and achieving goals. Choose rewards that align with your values and priorities, such as buying yourself a new workout outfit, indulging in a healthy meal at your favorite restaurant, or taking time to relax and pamper yourself.

- Share your success: Share your achievements with friends, family members, or online communities who can offer support, encouragement, and celebration. Celebrate your progress publicly to inspire others and build a sense of community around your intermittent fasting journey.

- Reflect on your journey: Take time to reflect on how far you've come since starting your intermittent fasting journey. Celebrate your growth, resilience, and perseverance in overcoming challenges and achieving your goals. Use this reflection as motivation to continue moving forward with confidence and determination.

By celebrating milestones and achievements, you can cultivate a sense of pride, satisfaction, and motivation to continue progressing on your intermittent fasting journey.

Long-term Maintenance Strategies

Maintaining your progress with intermittent fasting requires long-term commitment, consistency, and adherence to healthy habits. Consider implementing the following strategies for long-term maintenance:

- Establish sustainable habits: Focus on building sustainable habits that you can maintain for the long term, rather than relying on short-term solutions or restrictive diets. Incorporate intermittent fasting into your lifestyle in a way that feels enjoyable, manageable, and sustainable for you.
- Practice flexibility: Stay flexible and adaptable with your intermittent fasting approach, adjusting your plan as needed to accommodate changes in your schedule, preferences, or goals. Allow yourself the

flexibility to enjoy special occasions, holidays, or social events without guilt or restriction.

- Prioritize balance: Strive for balance in all areas of your life, including nutrition, exercise, sleep, stress management, and social connections. Prioritize self-care activities that nourish your mind, body, and spirit, and avoid extremes or rigid rules that may lead to burnout or disordered eating.

- Monitor progress and adjust as needed: Continue monitoring your progress, reassessing your goals, and making adjustments to your intermittent fasting plan as needed to support your evolving needs and priorities. Regularly evaluate your habits, behaviors, and outcomes, and make changes accordingly to maintain progress and prevent stagnation.

- Cultivate a supportive environment: Surround yourself with supportive individuals who encourage and uplift you on your intermittent fasting journey. Seek out friends, family members, or online communities who share similar goals and experiences and provide encouragement, accountability, and inspiration.

By implementing these long-term maintenance strategies, you can sustain your progress with intermittent fasting and enjoy the numerous health benefits it offers for years to come.

In conclusion, monitoring your progress is essential for achieving success with intermittent fasting and maintaining your health and well-being over the long term. By tracking key metrics, utilizing journals and apps for tracking, prioritizing regular health check-ups and assessments, adjusting your plan based on progress, celebrating milestones and achievements, and implementing long-term maintenance strategies, you can optimize your intermittent fasting journey and enjoy lasting health and vitality. Embrace the opportunity to monitor your progress, celebrate your successes, and continue thriving on your intermittent fasting journey towards a healthier, happier, and more fulfilling life.

Chapter 11

Special Considerations for Women Over 50

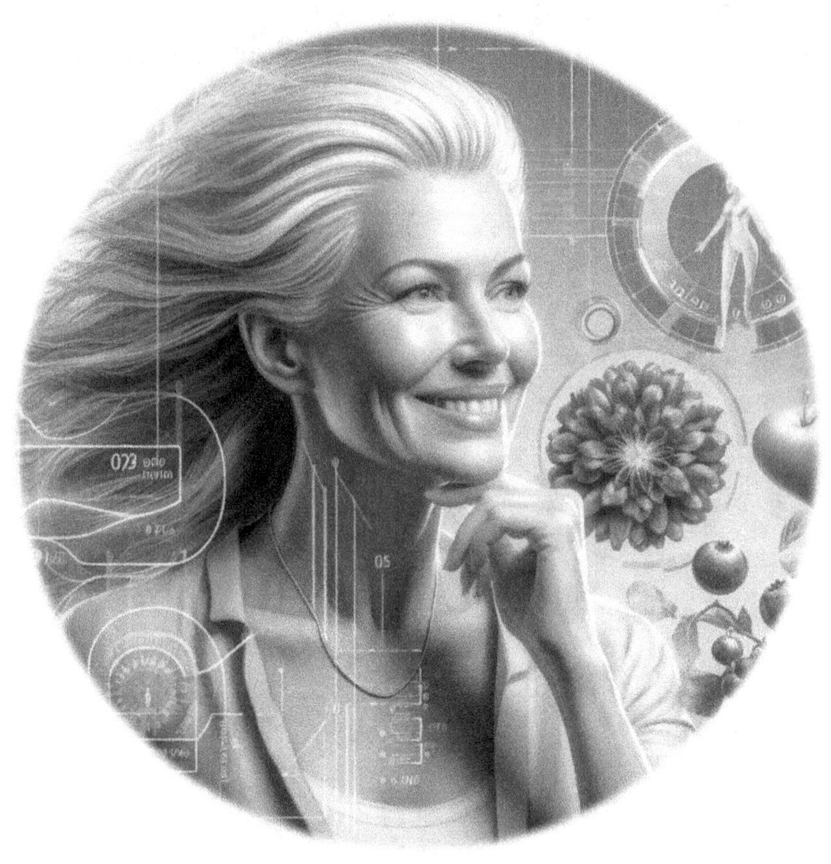

Women over 50 undergo unique physiological changes that can impact their experience with intermittent fasting. In this chapter, we'll explore the special considerations for women in this age group, including hormonal changes, menopause-related challenges, bone health and nutritional needs, managing mood swings and sleep disturbances, tailoring fasting plans for women's health, and personal stories from women over 50 navigating intermittent fasting.

Hormonal Changes and Their Impact on Fasting

Hormonal fluctuations are a hallmark of the menopausal transition, which typically occurs around age 50 for women. During menopause, estrogen and progesterone levels decline, leading to changes in metabolism, body composition, and overall health. These hormonal changes can impact how women respond to intermittent fasting:

- Metabolism: Estrogen plays a key role in regulating metabolism, and its decline during menopause can slow metabolic rate and alter fat distribution. Women may find that they need to adjust their fasting protocols or caloric intake to accommodate these changes and support weight management.

- Insulin Sensitivity: Hormonal fluctuations during menopause can affect insulin sensitivity and blood sugar regulation, increasing the risk of insulin resistance and metabolic disorders. Intermittent fasting may help improve insulin sensitivity and stabilize blood sugar levels in women over 50, but individual responses may vary.

- Appetite Regulation: Hormonal changes can influence appetite regulation, hunger cues, and cravings, making it challenging to adhere to fasting protocols. Women may experience increased hunger or food cravings during certain phases of the menstrual cycle or menopausal transition, requiring adjustments in fasting strategies to maintain adherence.

- Fatigue and Energy Levels: Fluctuating hormone levels can impact energy levels, mood, and cognitive function, leading to fatigue and brain fog in some women. Intermittent fasting may exacerbate these symptoms initially as the body adjusts to fasting, but improvements in energy and mental clarity are often reported once adaptation occurs.

By understanding how hormonal changes during menopause can impact fasting, women over 50 can tailor their fasting plans to accommodate their unique needs and optimize their health outcomes.

Addressing Menopause-related Challenges

Menopause brings a host of physical and emotional changes that can pose challenges for women over 50, including hot flashes, night sweats, mood swings, sleep disturbances, and vaginal dryness. Intermittent fasting may influence these symptoms in various ways:

- Hot Flashes and Night Sweats: Intermittent fasting has been shown to improve hot flashes and night sweats in some women by reducing inflammation and stabilizing hormone levels. However, fasting may exacerbate symptoms in others, particularly if blood sugar fluctuations trigger hormonal imbalances. Women should monitor their symptoms carefully and adjust their fasting plans accordingly.

- Mood Swings and Sleep Disturbances: Hormonal fluctuations during menopause can contribute to mood swings, irritability, anxiety, and sleep disturbances. While intermittent fasting has been associated with improvements in mood and sleep quality for some individuals, women may experience transient disruptions in mood and sleep patterns as their bodies adapt to fasting. Practicing stress management techniques, prioritizing sleep hygiene, and seeking support from healthcare professionals can help mitigate these challenges.

- Bone Health and Nutritional Needs: Women over

50 are at increased risk of osteoporosis and bone fractures due to declining estrogen levels and age-related changes in bone density. Adequate calcium, vitamin D, magnesium, and protein intake are essential for maintaining bone health and preventing osteoporosis. Women should prioritize nutrient-dense foods rich in these nutrients and consider supplementation if necessary. Intermittent fasting may enhance bone health by promoting autophagy, cellular repair, and bone remodeling processes, but further research is needed to elucidate its long-term effects on bone density and fracture risk in postmenopausal women.

- Heart Health: Menopause is associated with an increased risk of cardiovascular disease, including hypertension, dyslipidemia, and coronary artery disease. Intermittent fasting may improve cardiovascular health by reducing inflammation, oxidative stress, and risk factors for heart disease. However, women should consult with their healthcare providers before initiating fasting, especially if they have pre-existing heart conditions or risk factors.

Tailoring Fasting Plans for Women's Health

Women over 50 should approach intermittent fasting with caution and mindfulness, taking into account their unique physiological and hormonal changes.

Here are some tips for tailoring fasting plans for women's health:

- Start Slowly: Ease into intermittent fasting gradually, allowing your body time to adjust to fasting and monitoring your response closely. Begin with shorter fasting windows and gradually increase the duration as tolerated.

- Listen to Your Body: Pay attention to hunger cues, energy levels, mood, and other signs of well-being during fasting. If you experience discomfort or adverse effects, consider modifying your fasting plan or seeking guidance from a healthcare professional.

- Stay Hydrated: Drink plenty of water and electrolytes during fasting periods to stay hydrated and support electrolyte balance. Dehydration can exacerbate symptoms such as fatigue, headaches, and dizziness, so prioritize fluid intake throughout the day.

- Prioritize Nutrient-dense Foods: Focus on nutrient-dense, whole foods to meet your nutritional needs and support overall health. Include plenty of fruits, vegetables, lean proteins, healthy fats, and whole grains in your meals to ensure adequate intake of essential vitamins, minerals, and antioxidants.

- Consider Timing: Experiment with different fasting protocols and meal timing strategies to find what works best for your body. Some women may prefer shorter fasting windows or alternate-day fasting, while others may thrive with longer fasting periods. Listen to your body and adjust your plan accordingly.

- Seek Support: Don't hesitate to seek support from healthcare professionals, registered dietitians, or fasting experts who can provide guidance, support, and personalized recommendations based on your individual health needs and goals.

By tailoring fasting plans to accommodate their unique needs and preferences, women over 50 can reap the benefits of intermittent fasting while minimizing potential risks and optimizing their health outcomes.

Personal Stories from Women Over 50

Personal stories and experiences can provide valuable insights, inspiration, and encouragement for women over 50 embarking on their intermittent fasting journey. Consider sharing your own experiences, challenges, and successes with intermittent fasting and how it has impacted your health, well-being, and quality of life. By sharing your story, you can connect with others, offer support and encouragement, and foster a sense of community and solidarity among women navigating menopause and aging with intermittent fasting.

In conclusion, women over 50 face unique challenges and considerations when it comes to intermittent fasting, particularly during the menopausal transition. By understanding the impact of hormonal changes, addressing menopause-related challenges, prioritizing bone health and nutritional needs, managing mood swings and sleep disturbances, tailoring fasting plans for women's health, and sharing personal stories and experiences, women can navigate intermittent fasting with confidence and optimize their health outcomes in the second half of life. Embrace the opportunity to prioritize your health, well-being, and vitality through mindful and personalized intermittent fasting practices tailored to your unique needs and preferences.

Chapter 12

Special Considerations for Men Over 50

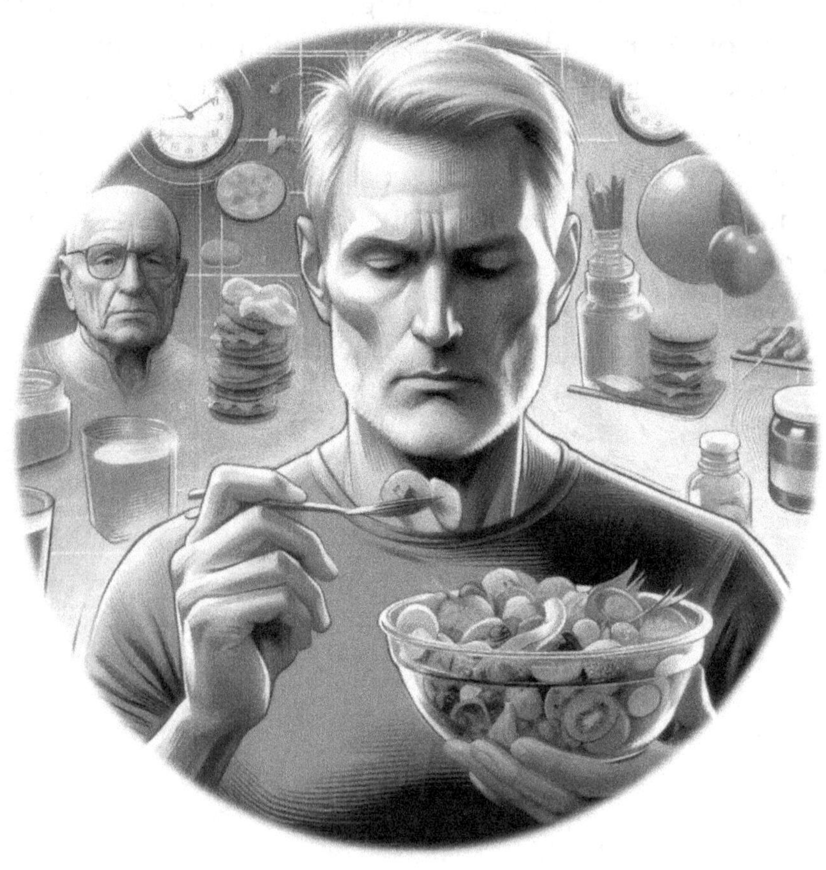

Intermittent fasting can offer numerous health benefits for men over 50, but it's essential to consider their unique physiological changes and health concerns. In this chapter, we'll explore the special considerations for men in this age group, including testosterone levels and their influence on fasting, heart health and metabolic syndrome, muscle mass maintenance and strength training, prostate health and dietary considerations, tailoring fasting plans for men's health, and personal stories from men over 50 navigating intermittent fasting.

Testosterone Levels and Their Influence on Fasting

Testosterone levels gradually decline with age, starting around the age of 30, but this decline becomes more pronounced in men over 50. Testosterone plays a crucial role in regulating metabolism, muscle mass, energy levels, and overall vitality. Intermittent fasting may influence testosterone levels in men over 50, with some research suggesting that fasting may temporarily increase testosterone production.

- Metabolism: Testosterone helps regulate metabolism and energy expenditure, and low testosterone levels can contribute to weight gain and metabolic dysfunction. Intermittent fasting may help improve insulin sensitivity, promote fat loss, and support metabolic health in men over 50 by optimizing hormone levels and metabolic function.

- Muscle Mass: Testosterone is essential for maintaining muscle mass, strength, and physical performance. Intermittent fasting combined with strength training can help preserve muscle mass and promote muscle growth in men over 50, enhancing overall strength, mobility, and functional capacity.

- Energy Levels: Testosterone influences energy levels, mood, and cognitive function, and low testosterone levels can lead to fatigue, low libido, and cognitive decline. Intermittent fasting may enhance energy levels, mental clarity, and libido in men over 50 by supporting hormone balance and metabolic function.

While intermittent fasting may offer benefits for testosterone levels and overall health in men over 50, individual responses may vary, and consulting with a healthcare professional is recommended before starting a fasting regimen.

Heart Health and Metabolic Syndrome

Men over 50 are at increased risk of heart disease, metabolic syndrome, hypertension, dyslipidemia, and other cardiovascular conditions. Intermittent fasting may help improve heart health and reduce cardiovascular risk factors by promoting weight loss, improving insulin sensitivity, reducing inflammation, and lowering blood pressure and cholesterol levels.

- Weight Management: Intermittent fasting can aid in weight management by promoting fat loss, reducing visceral fat, and preserving lean muscle mass. Maintaining a healthy weight is crucial for preventing metabolic syndrome and reducing the risk of heart disease and other chronic conditions.

- Blood Sugar Control: Intermittent fasting can improve insulin sensitivity, stabilize blood sugar levels, and reduce the risk of type 2 diabetes in men over 50. By optimizing insulin function and glucose metabolism, fasting may help prevent insulin resistance and metabolic dysfunction associated with metabolic syndrome.

- Cholesterol Levels: Intermittent fasting has been shown to lower LDL cholesterol, triglycerides, and other lipid markers associated with cardiovascular risk. By reducing cholesterol levels and improving lipid profiles, fasting may help protect against atherosclerosis and reduce the risk of heart attack and stroke in men over 50.

- Blood Pressure: Intermittent fasting can lower blood pressure and improve vascular function, reducing the risk of hypertension and cardiovascular disease. By promoting vascular health and reducing inflammation, fasting may help prevent hypertension and support overall heart health in men over 50.

While intermittent fasting may offer benefits for heart health and metabolic syndrome, men over 50 should consult with their healthcare providers before starting a fasting regimen, especially if they have pre-existing heart conditions or risk factors.

Muscle Mass Maintenance and Strength Training

Preserving muscle mass and strength becomes increasingly important for men over 50, as age-related muscle loss (sarcopenia) and decreased muscle strength can impact mobility, balance, and functional independence. Intermittent fasting combined with strength training can help preserve muscle mass, improve muscle function, and enhance overall physical performance in men over 50.

- Strength Training: Incorporate regular strength training exercises into your fitness routine to maintain muscle mass, increase strength, and improve functional capacity. Focus on compound exercises that target multiple muscle groups, such as squats, deadlifts, bench presses, rows, and overhead presses.

- Protein Intake: Ensure an adequate intake of high-quality protein to support muscle repair, growth, and recovery. Aim for a protein-rich diet containing lean meats, poultry, fish, eggs, dairy products, legumes, nuts, and seeds. Consider consuming protein-rich meals or snacks within your eating window to optimize muscle protein synthesis and recovery.

- Resistance Exercise: Incorporate resistance bands, bodyweight exercises, or free weights into your workouts to challenge your muscles and promote muscle growth. Focus on progressive overload, gradually increasing the intensity, volume, or resistance of your exercises over time to stimulate muscle adaptation and growth.

- Recovery and Rest: Allow sufficient time for rest and recovery between workouts to prevent overtraining and promote muscle repair and growth. Prioritize quality sleep, hydration, and nutrition to support recovery and optimize muscle recovery and adaptation.

By combining intermittent fasting with strength training, men over 50 can preserve muscle mass, improve strength, and enhance overall physical performance, supporting their long-term health and well-being.

Prostate Health and Dietary Considerations

Prostate health becomes a significant concern for men over 50, as the risk of prostate enlargement (benign prostatic hyperplasia) and prostate cancer increases with age. While intermittent fasting may offer potential benefits for prostate health, additional dietary considerations are essential for supporting prostate health and reducing the risk of prostate-related conditions.

- Anti-inflammatory Diet: Follow an anti-inflammatory diet rich in fruits, vegetables, whole grains, healthy fats, and lean proteins to reduce inflammation and support prostate health. Include foods rich in antioxidants, such as tomatoes, berries, cruciferous vegetables, nuts, and seeds, to protect against oxidative stress and inflammation.

- Omega-3 Fatty Acids: Incorporate omega-3 fatty acids from fatty fish (such as salmon, mackerel, and sardines), flaxseeds, chia seeds, walnuts, and hemp seeds into your diet to reduce inflammation and support prostate health. Omega-3 fatty acids have been shown to inhibit prostate cancer growth and improve prostate function in men over 50.

- Soy and Legumes: Include soy products (such as tofu, tempeh, and soy milk) and legumes (such as lentils, chickpeas, and beans) in your diet to support prostate health. Soy contains phytoestrogens called isoflavones, which may help reduce the risk of prostate cancer and alleviate symptoms of benign prostatic hyperplasia.

- Tomatoes and Lycopene: Consume tomatoes and tomato products, which are rich in lycopene, a potent antioxidant associated with a reduced risk of prostate cancer and improved prostate health. Cooked tomatoes, tomato sauce, and tomato paste are particularly high in lycopene and may offer greater benefits than raw tomatoes.

- Limit Red Meat and Processed Foods: Reduce your intake of red meat, processed meats, high-fat dairy products, and refined carbohydrates, which may increase inflammation and prostate cancer risk. Opt for lean protein sources, such as poultry, fish, tofu, and legumes, and choose whole, unprocessed foods whenever possible.

By incorporating these dietary considerations into your intermittent fasting plan, you can support prostate health, reduce inflammation, and reduce the risk of prostate-related conditions in men over 50.

Tailoring Fasting Plans for Men's Health

Men over 50 should tailor their intermittent fasting plans to accommodate their unique physiological changes, health concerns, and lifestyle factors. Here are some tips for tailoring fasting plans for men's health:

- Consult with Healthcare Providers: Before starting a fasting regimen, consult with your healthcare providers, including your primary care physician, cardiologist, and urologist, to ensure that fasting is safe and appropriate for your health status and medical history.

- Start Slowly: Ease into intermittent fasting gradually, allowing your body time to adjust to fasting and monitoring your response closely. Begin with shorter fasting windows and gradually increase the duration as tolerated, paying attention to hunger cues, energy levels, and overall well-being.

- Consider Hormonal Effects: Be mindful of the potential effects of fasting on hormone levels, including testosterone, cortisol, insulin, and thyroid hormones. Monitor your hormonal response to fasting and adjust your fasting plan as needed to support hormone balance and metabolic health.

- Prioritize Nutrient-Dense Foods: Focus on nutrient-dense, whole foods to meet your nutritional needs and support overall health. Include plenty of fruits, vegetables, whole grains, lean proteins, healthy fats, and legumes in your meals to ensure adequate intake of essential vitamins, minerals, and antioxidants.

- Stay Hydrated: Drink plenty of water and electrolytes during fasting periods to stay hydrated and support electrolyte balance. Dehydration can exacerbate symptoms such as fatigue, headaches, and dizziness, so prioritize fluid intake throughout the day.

- Incorporate Strength Training: Include regular strength training exercises in your fitness routine to preserve muscle mass, increase strength, and improve overall physical performance. Focus on compound exercises that target multiple muscle groups and progressively overload your muscles to stimulate growth and adaptation.

- Listen to Your Body: Pay attention to hunger cues, energy levels, mood, and other signs of well-being during fasting. If you experience discomfort or adverse effects, consider modifying your fasting plan or seeking guidance from a healthcare professional.

By tailoring fasting plans to accommodate their unique needs and preferences, men over 50 can optimize the benefits of intermittent fasting while minimizing potential risks and supporting their long-term health and well-being.

Personal Stories from Men Over 50

Personal stories and experiences can provide valuable insights, inspiration, and encouragement for men over 50 embarking on their intermittent fasting journey. Consider sharing your own experiences, challenges, and successes with intermittent fasting and how it has impacted your health, well-being, and quality of life. By sharing your story, you can connect with others, offer support and encouragement, and foster a sense of camaraderie and solidarity among men navigating aging with intermittent fasting.

In conclusion, men over 50 face unique considerations and challenges when it comes to intermittent fasting, including hormonal changes, heart health, muscle mass maintenance, prostate health, and dietary considerations. By understanding these factors and tailoring fasting plans to accommodate their unique needs and preferences, men can optimize the benefits of intermittent fasting while supporting their long-term health and well-being. Embrace the opportunity to prioritize your health, vitality, and longevity through mindful and personalized intermittent fasting practices tailored to your individual needs and goals.

Chapter 13

Intermittent Fasting and Chronic Conditions

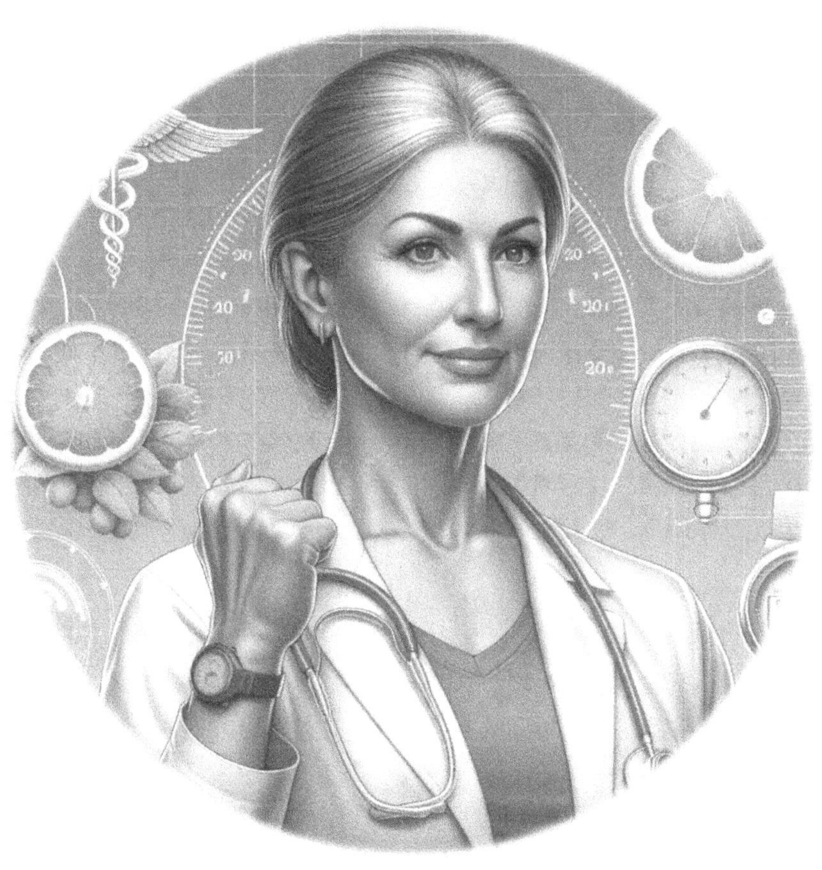

Intermittent fasting has gained popularity for its potential health benefits, but for individuals with chronic conditions, such as diabetes, cardiovascular diseases, digestive issues, autoimmune conditions, and inflammation, there are unique considerations to bear in mind. In this chapter, we'll explore how intermittent fasting can be approached while managing these chronic conditions, strategies for navigating fasting safely, when to seek medical advice, and success stories of individuals who have effectively managed their conditions through intermittent fasting.

Fasting with Diabetes and Insulin Resistance

For individuals with diabetes or insulin resistance, intermittent fasting can offer potential benefits for blood sugar control, insulin sensitivity, and weight management. However, fasting should be approached cautiously and under the guidance of a healthcare professional to minimize the risk of hypoglycemia (low blood sugar) and other complications.

- Consult with a Healthcare Professional: Before starting intermittent fasting, individuals with diabetes or insulin resistance should consult with their healthcare providers, including their primary care physician and endocrinologist, to ensure that fasting is safe and appropriate for their condition. Healthcare providers can provide personalized guidance, monitor progress, and adjust treatment plans as needed.

- Monitor Blood Sugar Levels: Regular monitoring of blood sugar levels is essential for individuals with diabetes or insulin resistance during fasting. Monitoring blood sugar levels before, during, and after fasting can help prevent hypoglycemia and hyperglycemia (high blood sugar) and guide adjustments in medication dosages or fasting protocols.

- Choose Fasting Protocols Carefully: Certain fasting protocols, such as time-restricted eating (e.g., 16:8 fasting) or modified fasting (e.g., fasting on alternate days), may be more suitable for individuals with diabetes or insulin resistance than prolonged fasting. It's important to work with a healthcare professional to determine the most appropriate fasting protocol based on individual health needs and goals.

- Stay Hydrated and Nourished: Adequate hydration and nutrient intake are essential during fasting, especially for individuals with diabetes or insulin resistance. Drinking plenty of water and consuming electrolytes can help prevent dehydration, while consuming nutrient-dense foods during eating windows can support overall health and well-being.

- Monitor Symptoms and Adjust as Needed: Pay

attention to symptoms such as dizziness, fatigue, weakness, or changes in mood during fasting. If you experience adverse effects, such as hypoglycemia or other complications, discontinue fasting and seek medical attention promptly.

By working closely with healthcare professionals and monitoring blood sugar levels regularly, individuals with diabetes or insulin resistance can safely incorporate intermittent fasting into their lifestyle to support blood sugar control, insulin sensitivity, and overall health.

Managing Cardiovascular Diseases

Intermittent fasting may offer potential benefits for managing cardiovascular diseases, such as hypertension, dyslipidemia, and coronary artery disease. However, individuals with cardiovascular diseases should approach fasting cautiously and under the guidance of a healthcare professional to minimize the risk of complications.

- Consult with a Cardiologist: Before starting intermittent fasting, individuals with cardiovascular diseases should consult with their cardiologists to ensure that fasting is safe and appropriate for their condition. Cardiologists can assess cardiovascular risk factors, monitor cardiac function, and provide personalized recommendations for fasting.

- Focus on Heart-healthy Eating: During eating windows, prioritize heart-healthy foods that support cardiovascular health, such as fruits, vegetables, whole grains, lean proteins, and healthy fats. Limiting sodium, saturated fats, trans fats, and cholesterol can help reduce the risk of hypertension, dyslipidemia, and other cardiovascular conditions.

- Monitor Blood Pressure and Lipid Levels: Regular monitoring of blood pressure, cholesterol levels, and other cardiovascular markers is essential for individuals with cardiovascular diseases during fasting. Monitoring these parameters can help assess cardiovascular risk, track progress, and guide adjustments in treatment plans or fasting protocols.

- Consider Medication Timing: For individuals taking medications for cardiovascular diseases, timing medication doses with eating windows or non-fasting periods may be necessary to optimize therapeutic effects and minimize side effects. Consult with a healthcare professional for guidance on medication management during fasting.

- Listen to Your Body: Pay attention to symptoms such as chest pain, shortness of breath, palpitations, or dizziness during fasting. If you experience any concerning symptoms, discontinue fasting and seek medical attention promptly.

By collaborating with healthcare professionals, adopting heart-healthy eating habits, monitoring cardiovascular markers regularly, and listening to their bodies, individuals with cardiovascular diseases can safely incorporate intermittent fasting into their lifestyle to support heart health and overall well-being.

Fasting and Digestive Health

Intermittent fasting may have implications for digestive health, including gastrointestinal function, gut microbiota composition, and digestive disorders such as irritable bowel syndrome (IBS) or gastroesophageal reflux disease (GERD). While some individuals may experience improvements in digestive symptoms with fasting, others may find that fasting exacerbates existing digestive issues.

- Assess Digestive Symptoms: Before starting intermittent fasting, individuals with digestive issues should assess their symptoms and consult with a gastroenterologist or healthcare professional to determine whether fasting is appropriate for their condition. Digestive symptoms such as abdominal pain, bloating, diarrhea, constipation, or reflux may warrant further evaluation and management before initiating fasting.

- Start Slowly and Gradually: Individuals with digestive issues should start intermittent fasting slowly and gradually, allowing their bodies time to adapt to fasting and monitoring their symptoms closely. Beginning with shorter fasting windows and gradually increasing the duration as tolerated can help minimize digestive discomfort and optimize adherence.

- Consider Fasting Protocols: Certain fasting protocols, such as time-restricted eating or modified fasting, may be more suitable for individuals with digestive issues than prolonged fasting or extended fasts. Experimenting with different fasting protocols and meal timing strategies can help identify the approach that best supports digestive health and symptom management.

- Prioritize Gut-friendly Foods: During eating windows, focus on consuming gut-friendly foods that support digestive health, such as fiber-rich fruits and vegetables, fermented foods, prebiotics, and probiotics. These foods can help promote a healthy gut microbiota, improve bowel regularity, and alleviate digestive symptoms.

- Stay Hydrated and Nourished: Adequate hydration and nutrient intake are essential for supporting digestive health during fasting. Drinking plenty of water and consuming electrolytes can help prevent dehydration and maintain optimal hydration levels, while consuming nutrient-dense foods during eating windows can provide essential vitamins, minerals, and antioxidants to support overall health.

By working closely with healthcare professionals, starting slowly and gradually, experimenting with different fasting protocols, prioritizing gut-friendly foods, and staying hydrated and nourished, individuals with digestive issues can safely incorporate intermittent fasting into their lifestyle to support digestive health and overall well-being.

Autoimmune Conditions and Inflammation

Intermittent fasting may have implications for autoimmune conditions, such as rheumatoid arthritis, lupus, multiple sclerosis, inflammatory bowel disease (IBD), psoriasis, and autoimmune thyroid disorders. While some research suggests that fasting may reduce inflammation and improve symptoms in autoimmune conditions, more studies are needed to understand the effects of fasting on immune function and autoimmune disease progression.

● Consult with a Rheumatologist or Immunologist:

Individuals with autoimmune conditions should consult with their rheumatologists, immunologists, or healthcare professionals before starting intermittent fasting to discuss the potential risks and benefits for their condition. Healthcare providers can provide personalized recommendations and monitor disease activity and symptoms during fasting.

- Monitor Disease Activity and Symptoms: Regular monitoring of disease activity, symptoms, and inflammatory markers is essential for individuals with autoimmune conditions during fasting. Monitoring disease activity can help assess treatment response, track changes in symptoms, and detect disease flares or exacerbations promptly.

- Consider Fasting Protocols: Certain fasting protocols, such as time-restricted eating or modified fasting, may be more suitable for individuals with autoimmune conditions than prolonged fasting or extended fasts. Experimenting with different fasting protocols and meal timing strategies can help identify the approach that best supports immune function and symptom management.

- Focus on Anti-inflammatory Foods: During eating windows, prioritize anti-inflammatory foods that support immune health and reduce inflammation, such as fruits, vegetables, whole grains, healthy fats, and omega-3 fatty acids. These foods can help modulate immune function, decrease inflammatory cytokines, and alleviate symptoms in autoimmune conditions.

- Listen to Your Body: Pay attention to symptoms such as joint pain, fatigue, rash, gastrointestinal symptoms, or other signs of disease activity during fasting. If you experience worsening symptoms or disease flares, discontinue fasting and consult with your healthcare provider for further evaluation and management.

By collaborating with healthcare professionals, monitoring disease activity and symptoms, experimenting with different fasting protocols, prioritizing anti-inflammatory foods, and listening to their bodies, individuals with autoimmune conditions can safely explore intermittent fasting as a potential adjunctive therapy to support immune health and symptom management.

When to Seek Medical Advice

While intermittent fasting can offer potential benefits for individuals with chronic conditions, it's essential to recognize when to seek medical advice or discontinue fasting. Here are some signs and symptoms that may indicate the need for medical evaluation during fasting:

- Severe Hypoglycemia: Symptoms such as dizziness, confusion, weakness, sweating, or fainting may indicate severe hypoglycemia and require immediate medical attention.

- Worsening of Chronic Conditions: If fasting exacerbates existing symptoms or leads to worsening of chronic conditions, such as diabetes, cardiovascular diseases, digestive issues, or autoimmune conditions, discontinue fasting and consult with a healthcare professional promptly.

- Unintended Weight Loss: Significant unintended weight loss during fasting may indicate malnutrition, dehydration, or underlying health issues and warrants medical evaluation.

- Persistent Symptoms: Persistent symptoms such as nausea, vomiting, diarrhea, abdominal pain, headache, fatigue, or mood changes during fasting may indicate underlying health problems and should be evaluated by a healthcare provider.

- Medication Adjustments: If you are taking medications for chronic conditions, consult with your healthcare provider before starting intermittent fasting to determine whether medication adjustments are necessary to prevent complications or adverse effects.

Success Stories of Individuals Managing Chronic Conditions

Despite the challenges, many individuals with chronic conditions have successfully incorporated intermittent fasting into their lifestyle and experienced improvements in their health and well-being. Here are some success stories of individuals who have effectively managed their chronic conditions through intermittent fasting:

- **Diabetes:** John, a 55-year-old man with type 2 diabetes, struggled to control his blood sugar levels despite medication and lifestyle modifications. After consulting with his healthcare provider, John started intermittent fasting with a 16:8 fasting protocol and noticed significant improvements in his blood sugar control, weight, and energy levels. With regular monitoring and support from his healthcare team, John has successfully managed his diabetes through intermittent fasting and enjoys a healthier, more active lifestyle.

- **Cardiovascular Diseases:** Sarah, a 60-year-old woman with hypertension and high cholesterol, was concerned about her risk of heart disease and stroke. With guidance from her cardiologist, Sarah adopted a time-restricted eating approach and focused on heart-healthy eating habits. Over time, Sarah experienced improvements in her blood pressure, cholesterol levels, and overall cardiovascular health. Today, Sarah enjoys better health and peace of mind, thanks to her commitment to intermittent fasting and lifestyle changes.

- **Digestive Issues:** Mike, a 50-year-old man with irritable bowel syndrome (IBS), struggled with abdominal pain, bloating, and diarrhea for years. After researching the potential benefits of intermittent fasting for digestive health, Mike decided to give it a try. With careful monitoring and support from his gastroenterologist, Mike started intermittent fasting with a modified fasting protocol and noticed significant improvements in his digestive symptoms. By prioritizing gut-friendly foods and staying hydrated during eating windows, Mike has successfully managed his IBS and enjoys a better quality of life.

- **Autoimmune Conditions:** Lisa, a 45-year-old woman with rheumatoid arthritis, experienced chronic joint pain, stiffness, and fatigue that affected her daily life. Determined to find relief, Lisa consulted with her rheumatologist and explored complementary approaches, including intermittent fasting. With guidance from her healthcare team, Lisa adopted a time-restricted eating approach and focused on anti-inflammatory foods. Over time, Lisa noticed improvements in her joint pain, fatigue, and overall well-being.

Today, Lisa continues to manage her rheumatoid arthritis through intermittent fasting and enjoys a more active and fulfilling lifestyle.

These success stories demonstrate the potential of intermittent fasting as a complementary approach for managing chronic conditions and improving health outcomes. By working closely with healthcare professionals, making informed decisions, and prioritizing self-care, individuals with chronic conditions can explore the benefits of intermittent fasting and achieve better health and well-being.

In conclusion, intermittent fasting can be a valuable tool for managing chronic conditions such as diabetes, cardiovascular diseases, digestive issues, autoimmune conditions, and inflammation. By approaching fasting cautiously, collaborating with healthcare professionals, monitoring symptoms closely, and making informed decisions, individuals with chronic conditions can safely incorporate intermittent fasting into their lifestyle and experience improvements in their health and quality of life. Remember to listen to your body, prioritize self-care, and seek medical advice when needed to ensure a safe and successful fasting experience.

Chapter 14

Long-term Sustainability

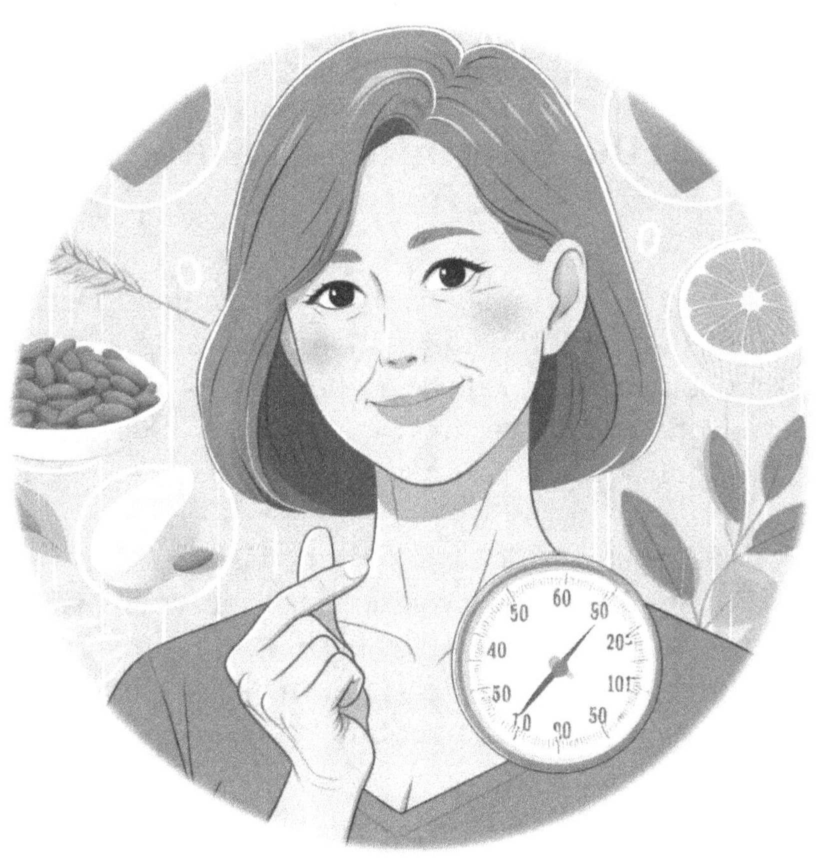

Intermittent fasting offers a promising approach to improving health and well-being, but its long-term sustainability depends on several factors, including making it a lifestyle, adapting your plan as you age, balancing flexibility and consistency, building a supportive community, continued education, and staying informed. In this chapter, we'll explore strategies for maintaining intermittent fasting as a sustainable lifestyle choice and accessing resources for ongoing support.

Making Intermittent Fasting a Lifestyle

The key to long-term success with intermittent fasting is to integrate it into your daily routine and make it a sustainable lifestyle choice rather than a short-term diet. Here are some tips for making intermittent fasting a lifestyle:

- Consistency: Stick to your fasting schedule consistently, aiming for regularity in your fasting and eating windows. Establishing a routine helps reinforce fasting habits and makes it easier to adhere to your plan over time.

- Mindful Eating: Practice mindful eating during your eating windows, focusing on nourishing your body with nutrient-dense foods and savoring each meal. Pay attention to hunger and fullness cues, and avoid overeating or mindless snacking.

- Flexibility: Be flexible and adaptable with your fasting plan, allowing for variations in your schedule, social events, or special occasions. Flexibility is essential for long-term sustainability and enables you to maintain a healthy balance between fasting and lifestyle preferences.

- Enjoyment: Find ways to make intermittent fasting enjoyable and rewarding, whether it's experimenting with new recipes, sharing meals with loved ones, or exploring different fasting protocols. Cultivate a positive attitude towards fasting and embrace the benefits it brings to your health and well-being.

- Self-Compassion: Be kind to yourself and practice self-compassion throughout your intermittent fasting journey. Accept that there will be ups and downs along the way, and focus on progress rather than perfection.

By incorporating intermittent fasting into your daily life with consistency, mindfulness, flexibility, enjoyment, and self-compassion, you can make it a sustainable lifestyle choice for long-term health and well-being.

Adapting Your Plan as You Age

As you age, your nutritional needs, lifestyle preferences, and health goals may evolve, requiring adjustments to your intermittent fasting plan. Here are some considerations for adapting your plan as you age:

- Metabolic Changes: Recognize that metabolic changes occur with age, affecting factors such as metabolism, hormone levels, muscle mass, and energy expenditure. Adjust your fasting protocol accordingly to accommodate these changes and support metabolic health.

- Nutritional Needs: Pay attention to your nutritional needs as you age, focusing on nutrient-dense foods that support overall health and vitality. Consider incorporating foods rich in vitamins, minerals, antioxidants, and essential nutrients into your meals to meet your changing nutritional requirements.

- Physical Activity: Stay physically active and engage in regular exercise to maintain muscle mass, strength, flexibility, and mobility as you age. Adapt your exercise routine to suit your abilities, preferences, and lifestyle, incorporating activities that you enjoy and that support your overall well-being.

- Health Considerations: Be mindful of any health conditions or concerns that may arise with age and consult with healthcare professionals as needed to address them. Adjust your fasting plan to accommodate any medical advice or treatment recommendations and prioritize your health and safety.

- Lifestyle Factors: Take into account changes in lifestyle factors such as work, family commitments, social activities, and leisure pursuits as you age. Modify your fasting plan to fit your current lifestyle and ensure that it remains sustainable and enjoyable.

By staying attuned to your body's changing needs and adapting your intermittent fasting plan accordingly, you can continue to derive benefits from fasting while aging gracefully and maintaining optimal health and well-being.

Balancing Flexibility and Consistency

Achieving long-term sustainability with intermittent fasting requires striking a balance between flexibility and consistency in your approach. Here's how to find the right balance:

- Set Realistic Goals: Establish achievable goals that align with your lifestyle, preferences, and health objectives. Break down your goals into manageable steps and celebrate your progress along the way.

- Be Flexible: Allow for flexibility in your fasting plan to accommodate variations in your schedule, social commitments, travel, and special occasions. Flexibility enables you to maintain consistency over the long term without feeling deprived or restricted.

- Stay Consistent: Maintain consistency with your fasting schedule and eating habits to establish sustainable routines and reinforce positive behaviors. Consistency is key to long-term success with intermittent fasting and ensures that you stay on track with your health goals.

- Listen to Your Body: Pay attention to your body's cues and signals, adjusting your fasting plan as needed to support your physical, mental, and emotional well-being. Trust your instincts and honor your body's needs, whether it's hunger, fatigue, or rest.

- Practice Self-Care: Prioritize self-care practices such as adequate sleep, stress management, relaxation techniques, and self-reflection to maintain balance and harmony in your life. Nurturing your mind, body, and spirit enhances your resilience and fortifies your commitment to intermittent fasting.

By striking a balance between flexibility and consistency in your approach to intermittent fasting, you can sustainably incorporate fasting into your lifestyle and reap its myriad benefits for long-term health and well-being.

Building a Supportive Community

A supportive community can be instrumental in sustaining your intermittent fasting journey and providing encouragement, accountability, and motivation along the way. Here's how to build a supportive community:

- Connect with Like-minded Individuals: Seek out individuals who share your interest in intermittent fasting and join online forums, social media groups, or local meetups to connect with like-minded individuals. Sharing experiences, tips, and resources with others can foster a sense of camaraderie and support.

- Involve Friends and Family: Share your intermittent fasting journey with friends and family members who are supportive of your goals and aspirations. Engage them in meal planning, recipe exchanges, or fasting challenges to involve them in your journey and strengthen your support network.

- Find an Accountability Partner: Pair up with an accountability partner or fasting buddy who can help keep you motivated, accountable, and on track with your fasting goals. Regular check-ins, shared milestones, and mutual encouragement can enhance your commitment and adherence to intermittent fasting.

- Seek Professional Support: Consult with healthcare professionals, registered dietitians, or fasting experts who can provide guidance, support, and personalized recommendations based on your individual health needs and goals. Professional support can enhance your confidence and competence in navigating intermittent fasting safely and effectively.

- Share Your Successes and Challenges: Be open and transparent about your intermittent fasting journey, sharing your successes, challenges, and lessons learned with others. By sharing your experiences authentically, you can inspire, motivate, and empower others to embark on their own fasting journey with confidence and determination.

By building a supportive community of like-minded individuals, friends, family members, accountability partners, and healthcare professionals, you can create a nurturing environment that fosters growth, resilience, and success in your intermittent fasting journey.

Continued Education and Staying Informed

Staying informed and educated about intermittent fasting, nutrition, health, and wellness is essential for maintaining long-term sustainability and optimizing your fasting experience. Here's how to stay informed:

- Read Books and Articles: Explore books, articles,

research papers, and online resources about intermittent fasting, nutrition, and related topics to deepen your understanding and expand your knowledge base.

- Follow Experts and Thought Leaders: Follow reputable experts, thought leaders, and influencers in the fields of intermittent fasting, nutrition, and health on social media, blogs, podcasts, and other platforms. Stay updated on the latest research, trends, and developments in the field.

- Attend Workshops and Seminars: Participate in workshops, seminars, webinars, conferences, and educational events focused on intermittent fasting, nutrition, and wellness. Engage with experts, ask questions, and network with fellow enthusiasts to enhance your learning experience.

- Join Online Courses and Programs: Enroll in online courses, coaching programs, or certification courses on intermittent fasting, nutrition, and lifestyle medicine to deepen your knowledge and skills. Structured educational programs provide valuable insights, practical strategies, and ongoing support for sustainable behavior change.

- Listen to Podcasts and Interviews: Tune in to podcasts, interviews, and panel discussions featuring experts and practitioners in the fields of intermittent fasting, nutrition, and health. Listen to diverse perspectives, learn from others' experiences, and gain inspiration and motivation for your fasting journey.

By prioritizing continued education, staying informed about the latest research and developments, and engaging with experts and thought leaders, you can enhance your knowledge, skills, and confidence in navigating intermittent fasting and maintaining long-term sustainability.

Resources for Ongoing Support

Accessing reliable resources and support networks is essential for sustaining your intermittent fasting journey and overcoming challenges along the way. Here are some resources to consider:

- Books and Literature: Explore books, e-books, guides, and literature on intermittent fasting, nutrition, meal planning, recipes, and healthy lifestyle habits. Look for evidence-based resources written by reputable authors and experts in the field.

- Online Forums and Communities: Join online forums, social media groups, and communities dedicated to intermittent fasting, where you can connect with like-minded individuals, share experiences, ask questions, and seek support and encouragement.

- Mobile Apps and Tools: Use mobile apps, trackers,

and tools designed for intermittent fasting, meal tracking, hydration monitoring, and fitness tracking. These apps can help you stay organized, track progress, set goals, and stay motivated on your fasting journey.

- Professional Support Services: Seek guidance and support from healthcare professionals, registered dietitians, nutritionists, and fasting experts who can provide personalized recommendations, address specific health concerns, and offer ongoing support and accountability.

- Educational Programs and Courses: Enroll in online courses, coaching programs, workshops, or seminars focused on intermittent fasting, nutrition, and lifestyle medicine. These educational programs provide structured guidance, practical strategies, and community support for sustainable behavior change.

- Podcasts and Webinars: Listen to podcasts, webinars, and online presentations featuring experts and thought leaders in the fields of intermittent fasting, nutrition, health, and wellness. Stay informed about the latest research, trends, and insights in the field.

By accessing reliable resources, engaging with supportive communities, seeking professional guidance, and prioritizing ongoing education, you can build a robust support network that empowers you to sustain your intermittent fasting journey and achieve long-term success in improving your health and well-being.

In conclusion, long-term sustainability with intermittent fasting requires a holistic approach that encompasses making it a lifestyle, adapting your plan as you age, balancing flexibility and consistency, building a supportive community, continued education, and accessing resources for ongoing support. By integrating these strategies into your intermittent fasting journey, you can cultivate habits that promote lasting health, vitality, and well-being for years to come. Remember to prioritize self-care, listen to your body, and celebrate your progress along the way as you embark on this transformative journey towards optimal health and wellness.

Chapter 15

The 21-Day Meal Plan

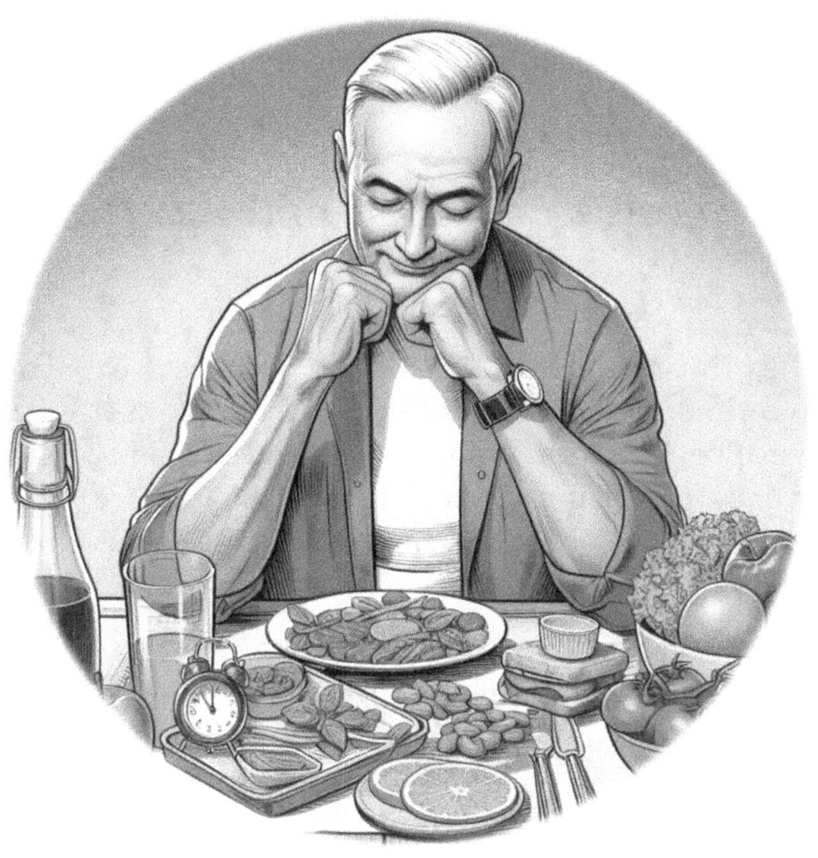

Embarking on a journey of intermittent fasting requires not just determination but also a well-structured plan to guide you through the process. The 21-day meal plan is designed to be your companion, providing you with a roadmap to navigate the challenges and reap the benefits of intermittent fasting. Let's dive deeper into each week of the meal plan and explore how it can help you achieve your health and wellness goals.

Overview and Goals of the 21-Day Meal Plan

The primary aim of the 21-day meal plan is to ease you into intermittent fasting gradually, optimize your nutrition, enhance your fitness levels, and foster overall well-being. Broken down into three distinct weeks, each phase of the meal plan focuses on different aspects of your fasting journey:

- **Week 1:** Adjusting to Fasting: This initial phase focuses on helping your body adapt to the fasting schedule while providing you with the necessary nutrients to sustain energy levels.

- **Week 2:** Optimizing Nutrition: During the second week, the emphasis is on incorporating nutrient-dense foods to support your health goals and balance your macronutrient intake.

- **Week 3:** Enhancing Fitness and Wellness: The final week is dedicated to integrating exercise with fasting and implementing strategies to support your mental and emotional well-being.

Let's delve into the details of each week and explore the daily meal examples, recipes, and tips provided to assist you throughout the meal plan.

Week 1: Adjusting to Fasting

In Week 1, your body is adapting to the fasting schedule, and it's crucial to support this transition with balanced meals and adequate hydration. Here's what you can expect during Week 1 of the meal plan:

- **Daily Meal Examples and Recipes:** Each day of Week 1 features a variety of balanced meal examples and simple recipes designed to provide you with essential nutrients while respecting your fasting windows. These meals include a combination of lean proteins, healthy fats, complex carbohydrates, and fiber-rich foods to keep you feeling satisfied and energized throughout the day.

- **Tips for Managing Hunger and Energy:** Throughout Week 1, you'll receive practical tips and strategies for managing hunger and maintaining energy levels during fasting periods. These tips may include staying hydrated, consuming high-fiber foods to promote satiety, and incorporating small, frequent meals during your eating window to prevent overeating.

By following the meal plan and implementing the provided tips, you'll ease into intermittent fasting gradually and set the stage for continued success in the weeks ahead.

Week 2: Optimizing Nutrition

In Week 2, the focus shifts to optimizing your nutritional intake by prioritizing nutrient-dense foods and achieving a balance of macronutrients and micronutrients. Here's what Week 2 entails:

- **Incorporating Nutrient-Dense Foods:** The meal plan for Week 2 emphasizes whole, minimally processed foods such as fruits, vegetables, lean proteins, whole grains, and healthy fats. These nutrient-dense foods provide essential vitamins, minerals, antioxidants, and phytonutrients to support overall health and well-being.

- **Balancing Macronutrients and Micronutrients:** Throughout Week 2, you'll learn how to balance your macronutrient intake (carbohydrates, protein, and fat) to meet your energy needs and support your fasting goals. Additionally, you'll focus on incorporating micronutrient-rich foods to ensure you're meeting your daily requirements for vitamins, minerals, and other essential nutrients.

By prioritizing nutrient-dense foods and achieving a balanced diet, you'll optimize your nutritional intake and lay the foundation for sustained health and vitality.

Week 3: Enhancing Fitness and Wellness

In the final week of the meal plan, the focus shifts to enhancing fitness and wellness by integrating exercise with fasting and implementing strategies to support mental and emotional well-being. Here's what Week 3 encompasses:

- **Integrating Exercise with Fasting:** Week 3 encourages you to incorporate physical activity and exercise into your daily routine while fasting. You'll receive guidance on the types of exercises that complement fasting, along with tips for timing your workouts to align with your fasting schedule.

- **Mental and Emotional Well-being Practices:** Throughout Week 3, you'll explore practices such as mindfulness, meditation, and stress management techniques to support your mental and emotional well-being during fasting. These practices help cultivate a positive mindset, reduce stress levels, and enhance your resilience in the face of challenges.

By integrating exercise with fasting and prioritizing mental and emotional well-being practices, you'll experience holistic benefits that extend beyond physical health and support your overall wellness journey.

Shopping Lists and Meal Prep Tips

In addition to daily meal examples and recipes, the meal plan provides comprehensive shopping lists and meal prep tips to streamline your grocery shopping and preparation process. These resources help you plan and prepare your meals in advance, saving time and ensuring you have everything you need to stay on track with your fasting goals.

Adapting the Meal Plan to Your Preferences

While the meal plan offers structured guidance and recommendations, it's essential to adapt it to your individual preferences, dietary needs, and lifestyle. Whether you have specific dietary preferences, food intolerances, or cultural considerations, you can customize the meal plan to suit your unique requirements while still adhering to your fasting schedule.

Reflecting on Progress and Making Adjustments

Throughout the 21-day meal plan, you'll have opportunities to reflect on your progress, celebrate your achievements, and make any necessary adjustments to your fasting routine or dietary choices. Regular self-reflection allows you to assess what's working well for you and identify areas where you may need additional support or guidance.

By actively engaging with the meal plan, reflecting on your progress, and making adjustments as needed, you'll set yourself up for long-term success with intermittent fasting and achieve your health and wellness goals.

In conclusion, the 21-day meal plan serves as a valuable tool to support you on your intermittent fasting journey, providing structure, guidance, and resources to help you navigate the challenges and reap the rewards of fasting. By following the meal plan, incorporating provided tips and resources, and adapting it to your individual needs and preferences, you'll develop sustainable habits that promote long-term health, vitality, and well-being.

CONCLUSION

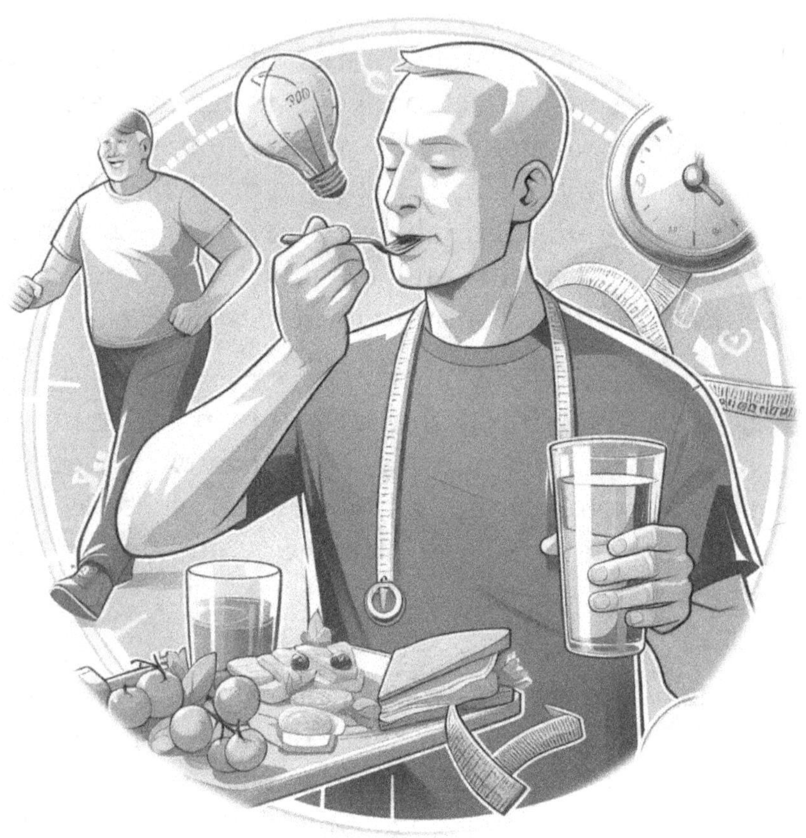

As we draw to the conclusion of this guide, it's crucial to reflect on the transformative journey you're embarking on and to reinforce the key principles and benefits of intermittent fasting for individuals over 50. Let's delve deeper into the recap of key takeaways, offer encouragement for your continued journey, explore the long-term benefits of intermittent fasting, share inspirational success stories, and provide final tips for sustained success.

Recap of Key Takeaways

Throughout this comprehensive guide, we've journeyed through the principles, benefits, and practical strategies of intermittent fasting tailored for individuals over 50. Here's a recap of the key takeaways:

- Intermittent fasting is a versatile approach to health and wellness, offering various fasting protocols to suit individual preferences and lifestyles.
- The science behind intermittent fasting underscores its efficacy in promoting metabolic health, reducing inflammation, and supporting cellular repair processes, particularly beneficial for aging bodies.
- Starting intermittent fasting involves careful planning, consultation with healthcare professionals, and gradual implementation to ensure a smooth transition.

Encouragement to Continue the Journey

As you embark on your intermittent fasting journey, remember that transformation takes time and commitment. Embrace the challenges, celebrate the victories, and stay steadfast in your dedication to improving your health and well-being. Each step you take brings you closer to your goals, and with perseverance, you'll reap the rewards of your efforts.

Long-term Benefits of Intermittent Fasting

Intermittent fasting offers a multitude of long-term benefits that extend beyond weight loss. By integrating fasting into your lifestyle, you're investing in your future health and vitality. Some enduring benefits include:

- Enhanced metabolic health and insulin sensitivity, crucial for managing age-related changes in metabolism.
- Improved cardiovascular function, contributing to a reduced risk of chronic diseases such as heart disease and stroke.
- Heightened mental clarity, cognitive function, and mood stability, fostering overall cognitive health and emotional well-being.
- Longevity and anti-aging benefits through cellular rejuvenation and repair, promoting longevity and preserving youthful vitality.
- Sustainable weight management and body composition optimization, supporting healthy aging and quality of life.

With each passing day of intermittent fasting, you're nurturing a healthier, more resilient body that will serve you well in the years to come.

Inspirational Success Stories

Throughout this guide, you've encountered inspiring narratives of individuals who have experienced profound transformations through intermittent fasting. These stories serve as powerful reminders of the potential for change and growth that lies within each of us. Draw inspiration from these journeys, knowing that you too have the power to rewrite your health story and create the life you desire.

Final Tips for Sustained Success

As you continue your intermittent fasting journey, here are some final tips to support your ongoing success:

- Stay hydrated: Hydration is key to supporting overall health and curbing hunger during fasting periods. Aim to drink plenty of water throughout the day.
- Prioritize nutrient-dense foods: Focus on incorporating whole, minimally processed foods into your diet to ensure you're meeting your nutritional needs and supporting your overall health.
- Listen to your body: Pay attention to hunger cues, energy levels, and overall well-being, and adjust your fasting schedule or dietary choices accordingly.
- Seek support: Surround yourself with a supportive

community of friends, family, or fellow fasting enthusiasts who can offer encouragement, accountability, and camaraderie on your journey.

- Practice self-care: Remember to prioritize self-care activities such as exercise, relaxation, and stress management to nurture your physical, mental, and emotional well-being.

By embracing these tips and staying true to your commitment to intermittent fasting, you'll continue to experience positive changes in your health and well-being over time.

Embracing a Lifetime of Health

In conclusion, intermittent fasting isn't just a temporary fix—it's a lifestyle choice that can pave the way for a lifetime of health, vitality, and longevity. By incorporating intermittent fasting into your routine, you're investing in your future self and taking proactive steps to optimize your health and well-being as you age.

As you embark on this journey, remember that change is gradual, and every small step forward counts. Celebrate your progress, stay focused on your goals, and never underestimate the power of consistency and perseverance. Your commitment to intermittent fasting is a testament to your dedication to living your best life, and the benefits you'll reap along the way will be well worth the effort.

Here's to embracing a lifetime of health, vitality, and joy through intermittent fasting. May your journey be filled with growth, transformation, and abundant well-being. Cheers to the vibrant, resilient, and empowered version of yourself that awaits on the other side of this journey. You've got this!

ABOUT THE AUTHOR

Adeel Anjum is a visionary business leader with an illustrious career spanning over 20 years in strategic management and consulting. With a dynamic background that includes diverse industries such as sports retail, fashion retail, food retail, oil & gas, F&B, fitness & leisure, as well as technology & telecom retail, Adeel has amassed a wealth of experience and expertise in driving organizational success.

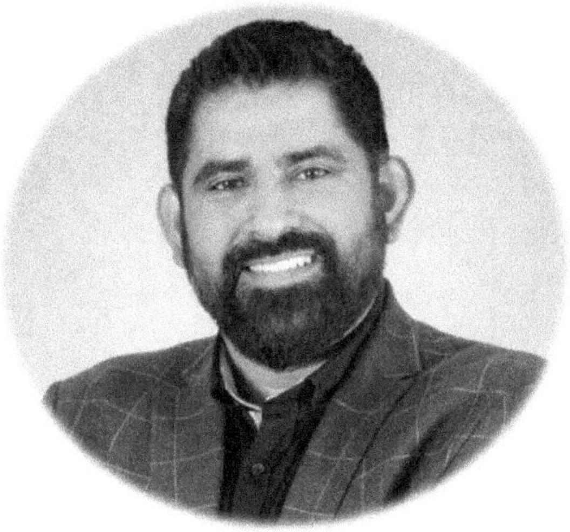

As a thought leader, Adeel Anjum stands at the forefront of shaping the business community through his pioneering work, insightful writings, and groundbreaking research. With a commitment to innovation and a deep understanding of Industry dynamics, Adeel Anjum inspires and guides fellow professionals, fostering a culture of continuous learning and strategic evolution within the business landscape.

Driven by a steadfast commitment to contribute to the business world, I am channeling my knowledge and experience into meaningful narratives within my books. My aim is to offer valuable insights, lessons, and strategies that empower individuals and organizations. Through the written word, I aspire to give back to the business community, sharing the wisdom gained on my journey and inspiring others to achieve their fullest potential and mindfulness..

www.ingramcontent.com/pod-product-compliance
Lightning Source LLC
Chambersburg PA
CBHW061638250726
48659CB00004B/1281